THE EMERGENCY DIARIES

THE EMERGENCY DIARIES

STORIES FROM DOCTORS INSIDE THE ER

NORTHWELL'S STATEN ISLAND UNIVERSITY HOSPITAL

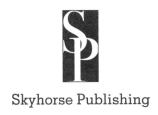

Skyhorse Publishing

Skyhorse Publishing books may be purchased in bulk at special discounts for sales promotion, corporate gifts, fund-raising, or educational purposes. Special editions can also be created to specifications. For details, contact the Special Sales Department, Skyhorse Publishing, 307 West 36th Street, 11th Floor, New York, NY 10018 or info@skyhorsepublishing.com.

Skyhorse® and Skyhorse Publishing® are registered trademarks of Skyhorse Publishing, Inc.®, a Delaware corporation.

Visit our website at www.skyhorsepublishing.com.

Please follow our publisher Tony Lyons on Instagram @tonylyonsisuncertain

10 9 8 7 6 5 4 3 2 1

Library of Congress Cataloging-in-Publication Data

Names: Staten Island University Hospital, issuing body. | Dowling, Michael J., author of foreword. | Brolic, Brahim. Telling someone they're dying.

Title: The emergency diaries : tales from doctors inside the ER / Staten Island University Hospital ; foreword by Michael J. Dowling. Description: New York, NY : Skyhorse Publishing, [2024] | Summary: "Harrowing and hopeful tales from doctors inside the emergency room at Staten Island University Hospital-one of the flagship hospitals of Northwell Health, New York's largest health care provider Open 24 hours a day, 365 days a year-through winter storms, hurricanes, and global   pandemics-emergency rooms are vital to the safety of any community. Day in and day out, thousands of patients pass through their doors to address their immediate medical needs. From life-threatening illnesses and injuries to sore throats and sliced fingers, ER doctors and nurses are the first line of defense when something goes wrong. Written as a series of essays and stories by real ER doctors, The Emergency Diaries gives readers a glimpse into the hearts and minds of medicine's finest, and the seemingly insurmountable challenges these everyday heroes face. Doctors recount firsthand the challenging nature of their profession and   the events that shaped their lives, and share pivotal moments in their medical careers that have stuck with them to this day. Whether it's delivering the bad news or making split-second decisions to save lives, the extremes of this profession can be overwhelming. ER doctors and nurses are under incredible pressure to act with grace, precision, and mental fortitude when caring for their patients. Larger national events-like the opioid epidemic, natural disasters, and the coronavirus pandemic-have only exacerbated this stress in recent years. This poignant yet hopeful book tells their stories, and serves"-- Provided by publisher.

Identifiers: LCCN 2024002603 (print) | LCCN 2024002604 (ebook) | ISBN 9781510778566 (hardcover) | ISBN 9781510781306 (ebook)
Subjects: LCSH: Emergency physicians--New York (State)--New York--Anecdotes. | Staten Island University Hospital--Anecdotes. | Hospitals--Emergency services--New York (State)--New York--Anecdotes.
Classification: LCC RC87 .E5255 2024 (print) | LCC RC87 (ebook) | DDC 616.02/50922747--dc23/eng/20240201
LC record available at https://lccn.loc.gov/2024002603
LC ebook record available at https://lccn.loc.gov/2024002604

Cover design by Kai Texel
Cover artwork by Getty Images

Printed in the United States of America

CONTENTS

FOREWORD

Michael Dowling, President & CEO, Northwell Health

They are the front doors of America's hospitals. Every year, emergency departments (EDs) throughout the country see more than 145 million patients seeking care for everything from life-threatening illnesses and injuries to sore throats and sliced fingers.

As New York State's largest health care provider, Northwell Health and the sixteen EDs we operate treat more than 825,000 emergency patients annually. About 125,000 of them come to Staten Island University Hospital's (SIUH) Ocean Breeze and Prince's Bay campuses, among the busiest within our health system.

Much like Staten Islanders themselves, whose neighborhoods, lifestyles, and viewpoints tend to differ from New Yorkers in the city's other four boroughs, the experiences of SIUH's emergency medicine physicians, nurses, and other staff vary in many ways.

During Superstorm Sandy in 2012, the surge sent water

lapping up against the doors of the hospital, but it remained open to those in need throughout the historic hurricane, recognizing the vital role it served in responding to a public health emergency that took the lives of twenty-four Staten Islanders, more victims than in any other borough.

Eight years later, those same dedicated individuals braved another public health crisis that struck Staten Island harder than anywhere in the city, with more than 2,700 local residents dying from COVID-19 in 2020 and the ensuing years.

Throughout the past decade, they've also seen the faces of countless others victimized by yet another public health epidemic that refuses to loosen its grip on our nation—the scourge of fentanyl-laced opioids that is killing more than one hundred thousand Americans a year, including 146 Staten Islanders in 2021—a rate higher than any borough except the Bronx.

Throughout the pages of this book, SIUH's emergency medicine physicians recount some of the many experiences that have shaped their lives, left an indelible mark on them as caregivers, and reaffirmed their commitment and dedication to their vocation.

We owe them—and the thousands of other emergency department professionals who come to work every day never knowing what they are going to encounter—an immense debt of gratitude. They are there for us twenty-four hours a day, 365 days a year, caring and consoling millions of individuals and family members during some of the most stressful times of their lives.

FOREWORD

I extend my thanks and appreciation to the SIUH team members who contributed to this book and wish them continued strength and perseverance as they heal and support their fellow New Yorkers.

THE EMERGENCY DIARIES

THE 2003 BLACKOUT

Dr. Yvonne Giunta

It was August 14, 2003. I vividly remember that day, not because of the way my day started, but because of the way my day evolved. At approximately 4 p.m., or 4:10 p.m. to be exact, one of the most memorable days of my career began.

I was still an intern with about two and a half more months to go before becoming a second-year pediatric senior resident. However, on that particular day, I was assigned as the senior resident in charge of the Neonatal Intensive Care Unit at SUNY Downstate Medical Center. So, there I was, an intern, acting as senior resident in charge of the NICU. Quite honestly, it was not a role I was afraid of playing. I just had no idea of the challenge and responsibility I was about to face.

In retrospect, it was better that I didn't know what was about to happen. Had I known, the panic would have likely crippled my brain.

At 4:10 p.m., in broad daylight, began the second most widespread blackout in history to date. It was a hot day, approximately eighty-eight degrees in Flatbush, Brooklyn. A software bug in the alarm system in the control room of First Energy was the cause. The outage, which spanned throughout the Northeast and Midwest United States and parts of Southeast Canada, lasted anywhere from two hours to four days, depending on the location. Fifty-five million people were affected, and approximately one hundred people died. While generators were clicking on all over the Northeast, at Downstate, the generators failed. My mind immediately went to 9/11. I didn't know initially what was happening, but the panic around me reminded me of that day vividly.

All our ventilators that relied on electricity weren't going to work. Our NICU babies relied on these ventilators. All our pumps that were plugged in would eventually run out of battery life and stop delivering fluids and medications. Our NICU babies needed these drips to provide antibiotics and nutrition. Luckily it was still daylight, but we weren't sure how long the blackout was going to last. Seconds turned into minutes. Minutes turned into hours. We needed a plan fast.

For over ten hours, the generators stayed silent. Yet, within the walls of this inner-city hospital in Brooklyn, there was anything but silence. We were the only hospital with extended power problems. Our backup generators failed, and until emergency generators were delivered, we ran the NICU with no electricity. We relied on battery life for hanging drips, our own hands to squeeze the bag and manually oxygenate patients in place of ventilators, and a lot of prayers.

Within the walls of the NICU, we had to figure out how

to keep our tiniest humans alive with no power. The day was a blur. What I recall most vividly was the way everyone pulled together to keep things flowing as smoothly as possible. The batteries on the pumps were not going to last forever. Oxygen in the tanks was going to eventually run out and we had no idea how long the blackout would last.

We plan for a lot of different scenarios and worst-case possibilities—fire drills, mass casualties, active shooters—but our generators failing is not something we typically think about. The generator is the backup plan. So, what happens when the backup plan fails? You are left with a night to remember forever.

We started brainstorming and came up with a solution, but logistically, we still had a problem. Downstate is located on Clarkson Avenue. Directly across the street is Kings County Hospital, which had no issues with its generators. Why two hospitals were built across from one another is still a mystery to me. Perhaps it was all designed with this particular day in mind, but likely not. The NICU in Downstate is on an upper floor. We had to get these babies down to the ground floor and across the street to safety.

On any other normal day (a day with electricity), if a patient needed to get from one hospital to the other, there was a formal process. This would occasionally happen if a test needed to be done at one facility that was not available at the other. Even though the two hospitals are directly across from each other, the transfer process for these tests involved paperwork, signatures, phone calls, sign-outs, and even an ambulance, just to cross the street. But on August 14th, there was no time or resources for any of that. In fact, it didn't even include elevators or traffic lights.

All types of hospital personnel came to help. Team members from security and dietary, nurses and doctors, all of us worked together. We took turns bagging; we came up with ideas, solutions, plans. Staff members managed to move these neonates, in their isolates, down flights of stairs and literally rolled the incubators across Clarkson Avenue while I stopped traffic. One by one, we moved six babies from Downstate to Kings County without consequence.

Once the transfer was completed, now hours into the blackout, we returned to a much quieter Downstate. We still had our less critical neonates to manage. We kept our step-down babies that we could safely manage in our dark unit. However, not even a blackout could prevent new deliveries. And so, like any other night, babies were born on this historical evening. All were delivered with no issues— except one.

What should have been a relatively simple call down to Labor and Delivery for a meconium-stained delivery, became our next NICU admission. Darkness was to blame. Anytime a baby is born, even if it's a full term, the NICU team is called to be at the bedside if there is concern of possible meconium aspiration. We must be ready in case the baby needs to be suctioned or given any sort of respiratory support. And so, with very little concern, and a flashlight, we reported to Labor and Delivery to assist as needed with the delivery.

The baby had a strong cry and perfect Apgar Scores. The

cord was clamped, then cut. Due to limited visibility in the darkness, the cord was accidentally cut above the umbilical clamp. The blood poured out of the umbilicus like a hose. The reality is that in a newborn even a small amount of blood is too much to lose. This full-term baby, who was otherwise in perfect condition, now needed to come up to our dark NICU. We needed to place an umbilical line, check bloodwork, give blood.

I placed the newborn on the warmer. We couldn't see anything, but we managed to place the umbilical line smoothly with the help of a flashlight. A beam of light pointed right over my shoulder at the newborn's umbilicus. The rest of the night was calm by comparison, a memory now lost over time.

Finally, at around 3 a.m., the hum of a generator was heard. Backup generators were delivered. By then, our sickest babies were moved out and our remaining babies were stable. Relatively speaking, it looked like we were having an easy night in the NICU. At 7 a.m., the next group of residents showed up to their shift. We met to do rounds and report on any events from the night before—a night for me that was like no other I had ever faced. Yet, there was barely anything left to show for all the work that was done.

The same resident, who signed out to me just twenty-four hours prior, was back for her next shift. She went home after her shift, slept the rest of the day and night away, and came in the next morning to a totally different unit, having no idea what we had just gone through. She asked me where all the babies were. Could my words do it any justice?

I can't exactly remember what my response may have been, but I can imagine the look on my face as I described the night I had just experienced. I wonder what we would have done had we not been fortunate to have another functioning NICU directly across the street. There may have been one hundred deaths nationally because of the blackout of 2003, but our six preemies thankfully were not a part of that statistic. The whole hospital pulled together for the sake of these tiny lives.

I feel that the best in people always comes out of need and wanting to help one another, especially when the lives of children are on the line.

I am not sure if their parents really understood what it took to keep them alive and get them the care they needed under the circumstances we were dealing with. I would love to meet those six humans today, who would now be almost twenty years old, and tell them this story.

ALWAYS ON CALL

Dr. Anna Van Tuyl

My critical care shift was the usual assortment of maladies: sepsis, STEMI, strokes, and the like. I concluded my shift and headed home on the Gowanus Expressway in Brooklyn. The Gowanus Expressway is a dark, winding, pot-hole riddled thoroughfare, which I use every day to commute to the hospital and back. This night was different. When I approached the Third Avenue exit, I realized something was amiss. I noticed cars were swerving to avoid an obstacle in the roadway.

As I drove slowly forward, I scanned for police cars, flares, or some sign of an accident. There was nothing. I finally came upon what I thought was debris laying on the roadway. Ahead of me was an FDNY ambulance blocking the right two lanes of the Gowanus Expressway facing the guardrail. There was another damaged car with an elderly couple sitting inside behind the ambulance. I thought they might have hit the ambulance, causing an accident.

What I thought was wreckage appeared to be a man lying

face down on the asphalt. I pulled my car over to the side of the road and without hesitation jumped out. I approached the man and turned him supine. I put my hand on the back of his head to turn him over and felt what I could only assume was brain in my hand. He had a faint pulse and agonal respirations.

I looked toward the back of the ambulance for assistance. Through the back windows, I saw another elderly woman facing toward me on a stretcher with an oxygen mask on. The two EMTs in the ambulance saw me in the roadway and began walking toward me with a quizzical look. I realized that they had not seen the man lying on the roadway, so I brought that to their attention. I couldn't understand why they weren't already aware of this situation. All three of us were confused as to what had transpired.

I assessed the situation. There were three elderly people (two sitting in a car, one in an ambulance); two EMTs; one perplexed doctor; and one man dying in the middle of the Gowanus Expressway; all while cars continued to drive past us. In retrospect, this was not a secure scene, but that was not my concern at the time.

I identified myself to the EMTs as an Emergency Medicine doctor. My scrubs gave my story plausibility. I explained to them that I found this young man in the middle of the road with significant head trauma and that I had turned him over. He still had a thready pulse but was unresponsive. I asked if they had the equipment necessary to intubate him. They ran back to the ambulance and returned with their bags, then questioned my ability to intubate under these circumstances. I confidently reassured them I was capable. With a flair for the dramatic, I stood up, threw off my bulky and now bloody winter coat, and proclaimed, "I can do this!"

It was dark and cold, and cars were swerving around me. I lacked the appropriate medical equipment, but what I did have was an overinflated arrogance which drove me to move ahead with this plan. There was no I.V., no medication, no monitor, or suction at hand. My "rapid sequence intubation check list" was not helpful in this scenario. I grabbed the laryngoscope and the endotracheal tube and forged ahead. I attempted to open the "patient's" mouth, but his jaw clamped down like a vice. Turning to the two EMTs, I sheepishly admitted I would not be able to intubate him. My ego deflated. (I often think if I had been able to successfully intubate him, this story would have had a much better outcome, but I am committed to the truth.)

The ambulance at the scene was disabled by the collision with the car and the guardrail. I asked the EMTs to call two additional ambulances—one for the patient in the back of their ambulance and one for the man in the roadway. Meanwhile, the EMTs retrieved a backboard and a neck collar from their ambulance to stabilize the spine of the man in the road. My coat was still laying on the ground, and by now my scrubs were covered in blood. Due to the heavy traffic, which was now building on our side of the expressway, the two additional ambulances were not able to reach us, so they approached from the opposite direction.

We had to lift the patient over the median that stood between us and the newly arrived ambulance, which was approximately five feet high, to get him to the two EMTs waiting on the other side. The challenge was to lift the backboard above our heads while trying to keep it level. His trip was a little shaky, but successful. The ambulance headed to the nearest trauma center. Lights and sirens. There I stood, in the middle of the highway. In the dark. Alone.

At this point, NYPD began arriving. None of the arriving police officers seemed interested in speaking to the woman wearing bloody scrubs standing in the middle lane of the Gowanus Expressway. In an anticlimactic fashion, I got in my car and drove home.

I was almost home when I remembered I left my favorite winter jacket laying in the middle of the roadway. Not ready to part with this article of clothing, I called the Director of EMS at my hospital and asked him to make a few phone calls to attempt to retrieve my jacket. After an hour or so, he called me back and told me one of the police officers would drop it off at the precinct near the scene of the accident. When I arrived at the precinct, I tried to explain my predicament to the desk officer. He didn't understand. And neither did the four other police officers I tried to explain this situation to. They couldn't understand why I would be trying to retrieve my bloody winter coat.

I had to wait several hours, freezing in my bloody scrubs. On one side of me was a highly intoxicated gentleman; on the other was a disheveled young man who had clearly been in an altercation. I sat there until the accident scene was cleared and one of the police officers returned to the precinct with my coat.

Several days later, after the police completed an investigation of the incident, I learned the facts of what had actually occurred that evening. Tragically, the young man I found lying in the road had attempted to commit suicide. He climbed onto the elevated section of the Gowanus Expressway and jumped in front of the car carrying the elderly couple. Their car swerved to avoid the man and hit the ambulance transporting another elderly person. The ambulance then hit the guardrail . . . just as I arrived.

I found out the young man died several days later, despite the heroic efforts of the team at the nearby trauma center. Looking back now at the events of that night, I feel sadness and frustration. Sadness because this young man felt that this leap onto the expressway was his only option; frustration that I wasn't able to save him. My years of finely honed knowledge, experience, and skill were useless in this scenario.

I often replay the scene in my mind and wonder if I could have done anything differently to save him. This is one of the most difficult challenges of emergency medicine; not knowing how our well-intentioned actions alter the patient's course. How much was predetermined before I even got involved? The doubt can be haunting and humbling. From my twenty-plus years of practicing emergency medicine, I have a collection of patients who float around in my head and will never leave me. Could I or should I have done something differently to get a better outcome?

The hope that I cling to is that these ghosts help me to be a better physician and a more insightful teacher.

BLACK ICE AND SILVER LININGS

Dr. James F. Kenny Jr.

Growing up, a steady stream of popular eighties movies were on the TV in my household. *Vice Versa* (1988) was a family favorite. The plot is fairly simple: a father and son magically switch bodies. Following one of these viewings, when I was about nine or ten, I remember my dad contemplating the havoc that would ensue if this supernatural mind-swap happened to us.

"You would have to be a doctor in the ER!" he said to me with a grin. "And I would get As on all your tests!"

My dad was an ER doctor at the hospital close to our house—the South campus of Staten Island University Hospital. As a kid, I remember going there more times than I can possibly count. By age eight, I knew the code to the ambulance bay. My sister and I frequently spent time there after school working on our homework in an old call room that had been turned into an office.

As I progressed through medical school and my Emergency Medicine residency, my dad and I would often talk about work. An interesting case here, a cool procedure there, we could exchange ER sagas for hours. It was, and continues to be, a unique bond. This connection was especially valuable during the spring of 2020 when COVID hit. At the time, I was in my second year as an attending physician at Columbia University Medical Center in Manhattan. With him being in Staten Island, both of our hospitals were at the epicenter of the outbreak.

As we fought through threats of no ventilators, insufficient PPE, and no obvious timeline for the pandemic to end, we leaned on each other for information and guidance as we both faced this disease for the first time. He had experienced and responded to other pandemics and disasters: HIV in the eighties, 9/11, Hurricane Sandy, and countless flu seasons. Despite all of this experience, a couple of weeks into the pandemic, he called me and underscored the magnitude of the situation and how unique it was.

"I have never seen anything like it. It is persistently relentless and unpredictable."

His tone over the phone was calm and matter of fact. Coming from a man who built a career being unphased by circumstances expected to make most people cringe, the solemn nature of his voice emphasized to me how profoundly impactful COVID had become.

This insight lent perspective to what was otherwise a chaotic time; it allowed me to grasp the novelty of the situation.

In medicine, we pride ourselves on having the solutions to problems, and it perplexes us when we don't. But even when that happens, there is usually someone around who knows how to respond. COVID was different. We were all in the same metaphorical boat, whether we had two years of experience or thirty.

In the ER, the strategy was simple: We prioritized teamwork and grit over everything else. We knew the frontlines needed help, so we worked with the hospital to redeploy people to assist. I'll never forget seeing a senior urologist help a nurse draw blood on a patient during that initial wave; this would otherwise be unheard of. We had broken down the usual silos that typically keep departments separate from one another and decided to work together. The unity that ensued was a positive light in an otherwise dark moment.

In early January of 2022, I was about two months into my new job at Staten Island University Hospital. It was a homecoming of sorts, seeing as I was born somewhere on the second floor. As I got out of bed on the morning of January 5th, I found myself in a familiar place: getting ready for a COVID conference call. In the twenty-two months that preceded this day, I had been on what felt like a thousand of these calls. This one was different. This call was scheduled in response to the Omicron wave. Omicron was the first variant since the initial wave that made ERs in New York City feel like COVID volume might overwhelm us again. In contrast to 2020, most of these COVID patients had mild symptoms, and some didn't have any—they just wanted testing.

Unfortunately, with limited venues available for testing on Staten Island, the ER was the main game in town.

As I scrolled through my phone to find the link for the meeting, I noticed a series of messages from my colleagues about "ice on the road" and that we may need to anticipate an influx of patients. Naturally, I looked out the window, but was surprised to see that life appeared relatively normal in Manhattan. Nonetheless, the focus of the call quickly shifted to the fact that twenty people had just checked in to the South-Site emergency department in the past thirty minutes, a number that was typically closer to three or four patients in that timeframe. Combined with COVID, the black ice had created a Mass Casualty Incident (MCI)-like event.

Knowing that I was scheduled to start my shift there at 4 p.m., I assumed this meant that I would be needed earlier and started to get ready. Before I could even find my scrub top, I got a call from our administrator-on-call asking, "Can you make it in by 1 p.m.?"

As I made my way toward Staten Island, the drive was fairly uneventful. The temperature was now over 32 degrees, leaving no trace of ice. I made a quick stop at our other hospital site to pick up my work phone, and on my way out, I ran into a coworker who knew I was working at the South site that day.

"Hey, you're heading to South, right?" he asked.

"Yeah, I'm on my way there now," I replied.

"Good, they need help down there," he uttered. "They currently have ninety-one patients."

The number seemed unfathomable. It was difficult to imagine that emergency room, which has about thirty-five "places" to see patients and a waiting room the size of a two-car garage, filled with that many people. Apparently, half of Staten Island had fallen that morning on their way to work.

As I got out of the car, I grabbed a mask from my backpack and quickly threw it on. Walking into the hospital, the first minute was calm and quiet. As I made my way through the halls, I noticed the security doors to the ER were open, and a wall of patients were sitting in a long hallway behind the ER. The anticipation that had been rising within me came crashing down and I quickly shifted my focus toward getting ready to see patients. I swiped into that same office where I used to do my homework, grabbed the rest of my gear, and headed toward the work room.

The hallway was littered with injured patients. Chairs were everywhere, leaving no resemblance to the usually organized room system. Many of the patients' eyes appeared anxious and scared; others simply weathered. Some had slings; others were bleeding from head wounds; a few had neck braces on. I passed several who were coughing and one or two that were clearly working hard to breathe as they clung onto oxygen masks. All this time, staff members buzzed around the unit with determination and focus, concentrated on completing their task.

Walking into the work room, I got the sense I was in a mini-command center. I was now the fourth attending (usually only two at this time of day), and there were four PAs (usually three). The phones were buzzing, and everyone had the same hyper-focused look in their eye. The scene felt familiar, and I was momentarily transported back to the initial surge in 2020.

At the front of the room, there was a senior physician communicating the severity of the situation to hospital leaders. He was explaining the need to label the hospital under a "disaster status." It was my dad. He had come in to help see patients on a day he wasn't scheduled to work. We raised our eyebrows to each other and smiled with our eyes while our faces were concealed by masks. Today, for the first time, we would be working side by side.

I sat down at one of the open computers and started assigning myself to patients. The first person I saw had a broken arm after falling in their driveway. The next was an elderly man on blood thinners who had slipped and hit his head. One of the other attendings had multiple patients with broken ribs and "popped" lungs requiring tubes to be placed in their chests.

As we all navigated through this maze of injured patients, trying to tease out who had serious injuries and who didn't, we had to have the same vigilance for the COVID patients. Most of them were there with "colds" and wanted testing, but occasionally, you would catch someone with low oxygen or trouble breathing. The situation was a little bit like playing goalie while the whole team is taking shots at you.

This trend continued into the evening. By now, we had

added a fifth attending to our crew. Over and over, we heard versions of the same story:

> "I slipped . . ."
> "I didn't see the ice."
> "I've been coughing since . . ."
> "My wrist hurts."
> "My cousin tested positive yesterday."
> "I landed on my hip."
> "The cut's still bleeding."

The next several hours were a blur of looking at x-rays, suturing wounds, and swabbing noses. We even set up a new system on the tracking board to designate which chairs the patients in the back hallway were sitting in. Occasionally, someone would say they came in for abdominal pain or chest pain, because, ultimately, other illnesses don't stop on account of an ice storm or a pandemic. Fortunately, though, because the temperature had risen above freezing by midday, the ice had largely melted, slowing down the flow of new injuries. Turning off this faucet was key, because the COVID patients continued to check in.

Slowly, but surely, we began to manage the surge, which was largely thanks to tremendous teamwork and support from the hospital. As I was scanning the hallway looking for a patient, I spotted one of the Associate Executive Directors of the hospital organizing chairs in the hallway. Later, I saw the Director of Radiology transporting patients to the X-ray and the CT scanner rooms. We never heard a raised voice from the staff, and there was more help than we could have asked for. In many ways, we had trained for this over the past two years. COVID, and its serial unpredictable surges, had provided us with the practice to rapidly coordinate efforts across multiple departments and band together.

What made this even more heartwarming was that the majority of the people working and helping were from this community. They were caring for their neighbors, and you could see that fact pushed them a little harder to get to the next patient. The patients themselves were also understanding. As if they had all been bonded together by this slippery experience, they were considerate of those sitting just a foot or two away from them.

As we started to get the ER census toward a more manageable number, extra staff started to wrap up their work and head home. After my dad had discharged his last patient, I tapped him on the shoulder and bid him farewell.

"That was the busiest I've ever seen it," he said.

To put this into perspective, his first shift in this emergency room was when I was about five weeks old. Never afraid to channel his flair for the dramatic, he simply followed that up with, "we were all gladiators today." To have finally worked as an ER doctor in "his" ER was surreal and special enough. But to also have the first time we worked alongside each other be one of the busiest shifts of his career, that made the moment even more memorable.

The South-Site ER ended up seeing 172 patients that day.

BLACK ICE AND SILVER LININGS

The usual average is about eighty-five. In the week or two following "The Ice Capades Day" (as it began to be referred to), I mulled over what he said at the end of the shift, and I couldn't help but reflect on what many of us have gone through over the past two years.

People who work in an ER are used to expecting the unexpected. We manage organized chaos and a busy work environment every day. But none of us could have ever predicted the turbulence that the COVID pandemic would produce. If you had told us back in March 2020 that two years later, we would hit record volumes largely due to another COVID wave, we wouldn't have believed it. Yet there we were, battling through Omicron and the result of black ice at dawn.

In the subsequent days, it was clear that our other hospital site was hit just as hard, as stories of people chipping in to aid the ER continued to surface. Amid an already intensifying moment in a drawn-out pandemic, many rose to the occasion to contribute to another "all-hands-on-deck" situation. Albeit still early in my career, I had experienced enough to recognize that this wasn't something to take for granted. Despite all the drawbacks of COVID on our healthcare system, it was clear that our ability to rapidly mobilize resources and support each other in times of need demonstrated a potential silver lining in the repeated crises we'd been forced to face.

When my dad started his career, emergency medicine was a fairly new specialty. He was part of a generation of physicians who fought to build its credibility to the rest of the medical community while they learned how to provide quality care to those with urgent problems. This cohort of physicians will always be considered heroic by the emergency physicians that follow them.

As I reflected on those who went above and beyond on "The Ice Capades Day" to help their colleagues and patients, despite everything they have endured since 2020, it demonstrated the perseverance and resolve of those who show up day after day to work in our ERs. The experience made me proud to work alongside a new generation of heroes—and at least one old one, too.

FIRST DEATH

Dr. Sarah Lee

"Excuse me, doctor, I think patient Miller just passed away."

My fingers paused over the keyboard, mid-sentence in the latest progress note.

"In room 24," said the nurse. "Could you call time of death?"

It was my second month of residency. I had moved—amidst a pandemic—halfway across the country to a new state to start work in a new hospital. After all, medical students are at the mercy of the "Match"—a nebulous process in which thousands of medical students around the country rank their desired residency programs and a computer algorithm determines where each of them ends up. It had plucked me out of the Midwest and dropped me into Staten Island, where I had never ventured to beyond my interview day and the free ferry ride during my last visit to New York City.

Orientation block flew by with its procedure boot camps, shadow shifts, and resident icebreakers. I was shy and unconfident. I knew these were my weaknesses from previous mentor feedback. But I had slowly been nurturing my self-confidence through the opening weeks. I was determined. I would not be the wallflower anymore. I was no longer a medical student and had to be the doctor now, if only the intern. My patients needed me to be competent and capable.

And yet, I blinked—and now I was the intern on call for the first time in the medical ICU.

"Patient Miller? In Room 24," the nurse repeated.

The nurse's words had left me stunned—but they seemed to pass unnoticed in the bustle of the unit. I squinted at my long patient list from rounds, littered with markings, lab results, and undone tasks. I remembered the little old lady we saw no more than three hours ago. I recalled gazing at her frail, tiny body and pale, listless face as I tried to communicate with her to no avail. She had a Do Not Resuscitate (DNR) order in red letters on the electronic medical record. I knew she was quite sick—but somehow the thought had not crossed my mind that this could happen so quickly.

"Room 24," a deeper voice now echoed. It was the senior resident on call with me, a third-year internal medicine resident. In my brain fog, I hadn't noticed his arrival. "Come, let's go," he said.

I followed him across the unit into the room. Ms. Miller was laying in the same position I had last seen her—face to the window, eyes closed. Her mouth was slightly open. I would have believed she merely fell asleep, if not for the asystolic line on her cardiac monitor.

FIRST DEATH

This was not the first time I had seen death—I had completed medical school rotation, after all, including several in the emergency department—but this was *my* first patient death as the doctor. And it floored me.

Doctors and other medical professionals have a more frequent and intense contact with death and dying compared to the rest of society; and yet, multiple studies on medical students' reaction to death show that most medical students feel inadequately prepared by their curricula for experiences related to end-of-life situations. Death is introduced early in our medical training inside the gross anatomy lab. The absence of any identifying features made those toiling hours spent in Anatomy Lab easier. Death had already taken its toll, and it left an empty husk where a person used to exist. After anatomy lab, however, there is little further exposure to the idea of death and dying.

There is even less practice in the skill of declaring a patient dead, as I suddenly realized.

"First, we need to check for reflexes," my senior resident said. "We generally use two—the corneal reflex and the gag reflex."

I watched silently as he performed both tests, all without a response.

"Now feel for a pulse," he directed me.

I nodded dumbly and placed my fingers on Ms. Miller's neck, waiting for signs of life ebbing underneath those vessels. A beat went by, and then another—I shook my head.

"Time of death: 18:28," my senior said. "Come, I'll show

you how to do the death packet. And we will have to call the family."

The next hour of tasks passed in a gray haze in my mind's eye—but with every subsequent task, one thought persisted: *Did we do anything wrong?*

A hundred what-ifs welled up inside me. Was there anything we could have done to prevent this death? To give this woman a little more time with her family? To keep her heart beating?

Modern medicine views death as something that can be resisted, if not avoided. This view of death is further compounded upon by society's tendency to delegate the responsibility of death to physicians. While it is widely accepted that death is inevitable, it is the doctor's task to ensure that the patient is as far removed from death as possible.

Novelist Rudyard Kipling once said in his address to medical students of Middlesex Hospital, "Death, as the senior practitioner, is always bound to win in the long run, but we noncombatants, we patients, console ourselves with the idea that it will be your business to make the best terms you can with Death on our behalf; to see how his attacks can best be delayed or diverted."

It is little wonder that, throughout medical education, death is continually seen as a failure.

Each one of us has ideas surrounding death. With my concentration on emergency medicine, I had always imagined death to be more dramatic than what I had just experienced. As a medical student, I witnessed numerous codes in bloody resuscitation bays. I performed CPR. I even intubated in my last emergency medicine rotation as a medical student. In my mind, I always pictured the healthcare team descending upon a stretcher, racing back and forth in a bright room—all working together to snatch the patient away from the jaws of death. In the emergency department, we always did everything in our power to save the person before us, to bring them back and get their heart beating again.

Yet my patient simply slipped away quietly, almost underhandedly. The way that she passed away seemed natural—as if she was merely entering an eternal sleep. Gone was the drama, the action, the struggle for life. In its place was a peaceful transition to the inevitable.

Ms. Miller gave me a reason to ponder, for the first time in my awfully young career, that perhaps death was not a failure of the team or of medicine—but rather a crucial part of being alive. As Yale professor and surgeon Sherwin Nuland wrote, "We die, in turn, so that others may live. The tragedy of a single individual becomes, in the balance of natural things, the triumph of ongoing life."

FROM PHYSICIAN TO PATIENT: REDISCOVERING HUMANITY IN MEDICINE'S CRUCIBLE

DR. NORMAN NG

Embarking on becoming a physician is an extraordinary odyssey encompassing a blend of scientific expertise, genuine empathy, and a profound understanding of the intricate human body. Amidst pursuing academic brilliance and procedural mastery, it is imperative to recognize the essence of human connection within this noble profession. My esteemed mentors have repeatedly emphasized the significance of genuinely comprehending patients' experiences and empathizing with their emotions, especially amid the tumultuous atmosphere of a bustling hospital. Ensuring their sense of safety and comfort should always be a fundamental responsibility.

As an emergency medicine physician, you witness patients during their most vulnerable moments and direst conditions. Establishing trust and rapport under such circumstances can prove remarkably challenging, as a doctor's primary focus naturally revolves around their recovery and alleviation of suffering. During my training, I, too, encountered instances where I became excessively engrossed in the physical aspects of patient care, unintentionally neglecting the humanistic dimension—the indispensable essence that guides their journey through the chaotic emergency department.

One day stands etched in my memory as the worst of my life—a day marked by exhaustion and the scars from incessant scratching. Weary and lying in the ER bed, an indescribable fear enveloped me. Oversleeping through my morning doctor's appointment, I attributed it to sheer fatigue from work. While absentmindedly brushing my teeth, I turned my head and caught sight of a lump on the left side of my neck. Initially, I attempted to convince myself that it was nothing more than a pulled muscle or a benign condition. But as I underwent an ultrasound, expecting a minor issue, a sinking feeling gripped my heart when the technician placed the probe on my neck. Weary and lying in the ER bed, an indescribable fear enveloped me. I quickly realized that the gravity of the situation far exceeded my initial expectations.

Swiftly, the technician summoned the radiologist, who urgently insisted on a full-body CAT scan and immediate follow-up examinations. Drawing upon my medical education, I understood that supraclavicular lymphadenopathy rarely bodes well. The realization dawned upon me that this could potentially be adenocarcinoma or lymphoma. Checking myself into the emergency department, a comprehensive scan of my entire body revealed a mediastinal mass with lung involvement and swollen supraclavicular lymph nodes. At that moment, I transitioned from being a physician to becoming a patient.

I still vividly remember the day after that fateful CT scan—I woke up uncertain of the future and where I would be in a few years. My career had reached a standstill, and my focus rapidly shifted from reading and practicing to uncertainty and fear. I got out of bed, kissed my wife, and walked my dog, trying to maintain a semblance of normalcy. However, I knew my entire life had been turned upside down. Despite reassurances from my loved ones that everything would be okay, it was difficult for me to internalize that thought.

Walking into the hospital to undergo my biopsy, I was met with gracious staff who took charge of my belongings and asked me to change into a gown. I spoke to the interventional radiologist who performed the biopsy on the suspicious lump in my neck. It was a moment of truth when I discovered the identity of my enemy and the formidable battle ahead. Although I knew, as a physician, that the procedure was perfectly safe and commonplace, I couldn't help but fear the worst once again. For the first time, I truly understood the immense fear many of my patients felt when they faced excruciating abdominal pain or the most unbearable headache of their lives.

Relief washed over me when the pathologist at the bedside mentioned that it appeared to be Hodgkin's lymphoma. While I didn't know much about lymphoma, I recalled from my medical training that Hodgkin's lymphoma was treatable and potentially curable. For the first time since I discovered the mass, I found solace and got a decent night's rest.

A few days later, I returned to work, attempting to resume my regular routine. However, with each patient I encountered, I saw a reflection of myself—the fear they carried as they walked into the emergency department, or lying in the hospital bed. Our roles seemed to have switched entirely in another dimension. I found myself dedicating more time to patients, genuinely listening to their stories, learning about their lives, and building trust with them. I realized that trusting a professional you have just met during the most challenging times of your life is a crucial aspect of healing, as the emotional support from the caregiver is equally as significant as the medical care provided.

Soon after, I had my first conversation with the oncologist. This experience brought me a sense of safety for the first time since that fateful day. The oncologist, a well-respected and highly skilled practitioner, exuded confidence that instilled a sense of security within me. As he reviewed my chart, he assured me that everything would be all right, and that this experience would become a mere blip in my life as I moved forward. Together, we explored several treatment plans, and he actively sought my input and thoughts, treating me as an equal partner in my own care, despite my lack of expertise in the field.

Subsequently, I received a stage 2 Hodgkin's lymphoma diagnosis, marking the commencement of my journey as a patient. A medical leave became necessary, abruptly halting the rhythm of my life. It was an immense challenge to shift my focus from the relentless pursuit of my career to prioritizing my own care and well-being. Since childhood, I had idolized doctors, perceiving them as superheroes—beacons of health—seemingly immune to illness. However, this experience shattered that illusion and emphasized the undeniable truth that doctors, too, are fallible human beings.

A year later, having emerged from the crucible of chemotherapy and radiation treatments, I gradually regained my health. Reflecting upon this experience, I realized that, as physicians, it is all too easy to lose sight of our individual identities as our careers consume us. We must hold on to our roles as human beings—cherishing our relationships as friends, spouses, and parents—and continue to engage in the activities that ignite our passions. Advancing in our careers should never entail sacrificing our multifaceted humanity.

Becoming a patient opened my heart to profound compassion and care, even if a physician may not fully comprehend the weight of a patient's fears. I now understand that every person who walks into the emergency department does so because they perceive it as a necessity, regardless of the severity or urgency of their condition. To them, it is a matter of paramount significance. For all the residents who may feel burned out, overworked, and jaded within the hospital environment, I implore you to remember that a twenty-five-year-old presenting with flu-like symptoms and a year of unrelenting fatigue may require more than just ibuprofen and a sick note. They seek our expertise and compassion, longing for reassurance and genuine care.

The lessons learned from being patients ourselves should serve as a constant reminder to devote time, understanding, and unwavering support to those who entrust us with their well-being. By recognizing the significance of the human connection in medicine, we can truly make a difference in the lives of our patients and offer them the compassionate care they deserve.

HUMILITY

Dr. Anand Swaminathan

Publisher's Note: (The names in this story have been changed to protect the identities of those involved.)

6:30 A.M.

Just an hour and a half from sign-out, the hardest part of a night shift. Since midnight, we've been elbow deep in blood, vomit, traumas, chest pain, and lacerations. Natural endorphins are spent. I grasp a large coffee, hoping it can get me through the end of the shift and the drive home. All the team wants now is a bit of peace and quiet to recover before signing out. My eyes close, just a bit.

Brrrriiiiiinnnnnnggggg!

The EMS phone ring pierces the lull.

"Dr. Swami, what you got for us?"

My hand reflexively pops up and grabs the receiver out of the cradle.

"Fifty-two-year-old man with syncope. No trauma. Was walking in Times Square with his family when he felt some discomfort in his back and passed out. Heart rate is 52, BP 74/42. Glucose is 132. He looks pretty pale. We should be there in about seven minutes."

Seven minutes may not seem like a lot of time, but there's a lot we can get done. I grab the residents and let the nurses know what's coming in, and that we need a resuscitation room and two nurses dedicated to the patient when he hits the door. Everyone puts on gloves and gowns as tasks are assigned: someone to start an IV, someone to manage the airway if needed, and so on.

The patient's low blood pressure (hypotension) and low-to-normal heart rate (bradycardia) is a concerning combination and somewhat narrows our focus as to what could be going on. Typically, the heart rate goes up when the blood pressure goes down. There are some toxicologic causes with specific medication overdoses, but the big cause ringing in our minds is blood in the abdomen. Bleeding in the abdomen can cause a reflex response that slows the heart rate despite the low blood pressure. In a man this age, coupled with the complaint of back pain, a ruptured abdominal aortic aneurysm (AAA) is near the top of the list.

We call the blood bank and request two units of unmatched blood as well as two units of plasma and let them know we may be calling back soon for a lot more. The ultrasound is placed at the bedside. If we're good, and a little lucky, we can see the problem immediately on ultrasound and quickly move from diagnosis to management. The mortality of a ruptured abdominal aortic aneurysm is over 90 percent, making every minute matter.

We hear the sirens and our senior resident, and I move to the ambulance bay to meet the EMS team and patient. They weren't kidding; he looks pale as a sheet.

"BP still 70s/40s. He's in and out, sometimes answering, and other times not. We tried but we couldn't get an IV in."

We run/walk the patient the fifty feet or so to the resuscitation room. Our senior resident directs one of the junior residents to put in a large central line, instead of bothering with an IV since EMS already failed. One of the interns grabs the intraosseous drill (which basically puts an IV directly into the bone) as a temporary vascular access for medications and blood. The nurses work like a well-oiled machine, getting blood products onto the rapid infuser. This resuscitation ballet is quite beautiful, but there's little time to appreciate it. I place the ultrasound probe on the patient's abdomen and it's immediately obvious that the patient does in fact have a ruptured abdominal aortic aneurysm with a belly full of blood.

"The patient has a ruptured AAA," I call out, "John, call the vascular attending now. Tell him we need him in the resuscitation bay. Amy, call blood bank back and activate the massive transfusion protocol and tell them we need another two units of red blood cells and plasma right away. Bill, go to the blood bank and get those units."

Seconds later, everyone is moving in different directions, carrying out their tasks.

"Doc, I've got Dr. B from vascular on the phone. She said she's literally walking into the hospital now."

Lucky for us; lucky for the patient.

"Hey Dr. B, it's Dr. Swami in the ED. I've got a fifty-two-year-old man here with a ruptured AAA. He syncopized in Times Square and came to us hypotensive and bradycardic. We've given him two units of packed cells, two units of plasma so far, and the blood pressure is the same. The ultrasound shows a large AAA with a ton of blood in the belly. Massive transfusion has been activated, but this guy needs the OR."

There was a pause, then I hung up the phone and turned to my staff.

"Dr. B will be here in two minutes. Let's get the patient on a portable monitor. Hang the rest of the blood on the rapid infuser. Amy, call the OR and let them know we're gonna be coming up in about five minutes."

Dr. B enters the resuscitation room a minute later, and quickly apprises the situation. We show her the ultrasound images and she agrees that the patient needs the OR. For a brief moment, my mind wanders and considers the fact that things never work out this way. The confluence of events that has taken us from EMS call to OR in about thirty-five minutes is incredible and rarely happens. As we start to roll out the door with the patient, it's like I'm already patting myself on the back: quick deployment of resources, logistical awareness, rapid diagnosis, aggressive resuscitation, and a surgical consultant to the bedside. I can't help but have a moment of pride.

Then, suddenly, the monitor flatlines, and the patient who was moaning a moment ago is completely still; he's in cardiac arrest.

A fleeting moment of triumph vanished.

We wheel him back the ten feet into the resuscitation bay, which is riddled with trash from all of the equipment we've opened and used. Amy starts compressions while John starts the process of intubation. Bill cracks the crash cart and grabs medications.

I turn to the vascular surgeon, "It's not gonna work. Compressions aren't gonna fix the rupture. He's just lost too much blood. I think we should open the chest and cross clamp the aorta."

The procedure I'm asking we do is called a resuscitative thoracotomy, and it is almost exclusively performed on patients who have a cardiac arrest or are near arrest after sustaining a traumatic injury (usually from a gunshot or stab wound). It's not a common procedure and it's definitely not something we would typically consider in a non-trauma situation but, in this case, it seemed to make sense.

Dr. B doesn't even acknowledge agreement. She's already asked Bill to get her a thoracotomy tray. A skilled surgeon wielding a scalpel is an impressive thing to see. Dr. B is in the chest in seconds and has her hand deep in the thoracic cavity locating the aorta. Within minutes, there's a clamp across the aorta and now, likely for the first time since the patient came in, the heart begins to fill with the blood we are pouring in. We administer a single dose of epinephrine directly into the myocardium of the heart and it's off beating again. The monitor shows a heart rate and a blood pressure. Dr. B's team has just arrived, and they wheel the patient toward the elevators.

The patient's family was just outside the room. I tell his wife what happened, what's going on, and that our team has bought him time to get to the OR and Dr. B's team is gonna do the rest. I let her know that he's obviously in critical condition but that we've given him the best chance for survival. She quickly thanks us, and we have a volunteer walk her up to the operating room waiting area.

7:30 A.M.

High-fives all around. It's a pretty amazing way to end the night. My coffee is cold, but who needs caffeine after that rush of adrenaline? Minutes later, during sign-out to the day team, we're already recounting the tale with only a slight amount of embellishment. We leave like conquering heroes, having snatched life from the jaws of death.

We were good. We were lucky.

11:30 P.M.

I'm walking back in. Feels like I just left. I stop by the hospital diner to grab a cup of coffee before sign-out rounds and I see the patient's wife sitting alone. I stroll over, as if I'm taking a victory lap.

"Hi. I'm Dr. Swami, we spoke this morning. I took care of your husband in the ED."

She's clearly quite distraught. I missed that when I spotted her from the counter. She says hello and tells me that her husband died this evening. They were able to repair the ruptured blood vessel, but his organs shut down and he had another cardiac arrest.

I'm shocked.

I shouldn't be. I know the mortality rate is extremely high, even if the patient gets to the OR, but I convinced myself that we had saved him.

I listen and tell her how sorry I am. She can't get any other words out. Her family has just walked in, and I take my cue to leave.

Medicine is humbling. Even when you know what's wrong, you know what to do and everything falls into place, things still don't end up the way you expect they will. These moments can destroy a clinician's confidence, their sense of self-worth, and their ability to practice medicine. Or, they can be the challenge that pushes us to explore our limits and find new ways to treat patients. Sharing these stories, while painful, helps us see our own vulnerability as well as that of those around us. It lets us see the commonness of how medicine humbles us.

MY FAMILY'S COVID STORY

Dr. Joseph Basile

Tuesday in late May of 2020. The concerned voice of an emergency medicine physician recounted an emotional experience that she had just gone through with a patient's daughter during the COVID crisis in New York.

The story was one that we have all been accustomed to experiencing firsthand in the hospital or hearing about in the news: Patients dying alone without being able to have family members bedside. At the end of the interview, the physician spoke about the importance of keeping our perspective and humanity during this pandemic, and not to only focus on the clinical medicine. The physician also ended the interview by stating they were planning on collecting "stories" from other emergency medicine physicians to share their experiences.

I broke down in tears when I started to remember my "story" over the past few months.

In the early spring of 2020, I was the Associate Chair of two emergency departments in New York City, which sees approximately 130,000 patients per year. My COVID story started in January/February 2020, like many other Americans, when I saw the stories coming out of China and Europe regarding the virus. Since I was involved in the administration of our department, there were a lot of meetings and planning of potential scenarios related to the virus. During this time, my thoughts on COVID at that time were more of a theoretical and potential scenario.

Then came March. Hospitals around New York City began to see COVID-positive patients. At this point, I knew it was just a matter of time before our hospital had our first COVID patient. In my mind, I thought it would be something we would have to deal with for a few weeks and then it would blow over. Even though we were all reading about the potential impact in areas like Italy, it was hard to wrap your head around what the local implications would be. We were optimistic that our healthcare system would be able to absorb this challenge.

I worked on creating a local model of potential hospital bed needs based on prior flu seasons, but because we were dealing with a new virus, our team knew these were simply hypothetical models and projections that were never put into practice. What we didn't realize at the time was that we were about to deal with volume and acuity that we could have never imagined.

The news came swiftly. We now had our first COVID-positive patient. At this point, everything changed. Our hospital opened a 24/7 command center. The laboratory testing protocols were changing what felt like daily. We were bombarded with challenges regarding appropriate PPE, isolation protocols, use of ancillary testing, staffing concerns, etc. Every hour or so we were hit with yet another question about how to deal with a seemingly "normal" topic in the past. However, in our new reality, we had to adjust and re-think how we operate.

In early March, the volume in the emergency department was normal and it was business as usual in the ED. There was a feeling that changes were coming, but no one really knew what these specific changes were. This was truly the calm before the storm.

By mid-March, COVID became personal. My uncle, who is an OB-GYN attending physician in the same hospital where I work, started to get a fever. Eventually, this evolved into daily fatigue and GI symptoms for the next eight days. The results for the COVID test took five days, but when it finally came back, we already knew what the result would be. I called my uncle daily and he assured me that he was doing "okay," just that he was tired and febrile.

After eight days, his daughter (my cousin) who is a nurse called me at work to see if she could bring him to the hospital because she was concerned about his hydration. He was able to drive himself to the hospital that day, so I was expecting him to come in for evaluation and maybe some IV fluids, and then I assumed he would be able to go home. When he arrived, I was called by the triage nurse who told me that his oxygen saturation was in the eighties. Then I knew there was a problem. I went to see my uncle and he looked tired. His oxygen was in the low nineties despite being on supplemental oxygen. His x-ray had classic COVID findings of bilateral ground-glass opacities, and he was admitted to the hospital where his oxygen requirements were continuing to increase. Within five hours, he went from driving himself to the hospital, walking in on his own, and not on oxygen, to being on a 100 percent oxygen non-rebreather.

Shortly thereafter, he was upgraded to the Intensive Care Unit. At this point, I stayed at his bedside for the next few hours, which were some of the hardest hours of my life. As an emergency medicine physician, I knew exactly what was going on and how this was going to play out. However, as a nephew, I remained hopeful that somehow things would be different.

My uncle was one of my role models growing up and we have a close relationship. He also has two twin sons who were resident physicians in NYC at the time. I was in constant communication with them over the phone because of the no-visitation policy in the hospital. Within two hours of being in the ICU, it became clear the direction this was going. At one point his oxygen level dropped to the fifties-sixties range. He was going to need to be on a ventilator. It was a surreal experience for me as I stood at his bedside holding his hand as anesthesia was called emergently to his bedside.

I have been present for hundreds of intubations in my lifetime, but never from this viewpoint. It was a scary, out-of-body experience. He was intubated successfully and placed on a ventilator. Then I had to make the difficult phone calls to family to update them. I stayed with my uncle in the ICU until late that night. As I walked around the floor, I realized that my uncle was "lucky" because he was able to have a family member present. All the other patients were unfortunately "alone" because of the zero-visitation policy. I was fortunate that I worked in the same hospital where my uncle was staying, so I could visit him multiple times per day. This afforded my family some comfort in knowing that a close relative was able to visit him.

My uncle is in his sixties and does have some medical problems, so we knew that there was a real risk that he potentially was not going to make it. The survival data at that time for COVID patients who required intubation was not good. We insisted on remaining positive.

After only being on the ventilator for two days, I received a text message from the intensive care physician stating that they were able to remove him from the ventilator. We were very fortunate. Although the odds were against him, he was able to get off the ventilator quickly and head toward recovery. He remained on high levels of oxygen in the ICU for the next few days and was eventually downgraded to a regular room and discharged home on oxygen.

Two days after my uncle was extubated and still in the ICU, I received a call from my mother that my ninety-year-old diabetic grandmother who lived alone had a fever. My mom visited my grandmother every day to bring her food and check on her. Since the pandemic started, my mom was extremely careful and would wear a mask and gloves when she would visit my grandmother. The only time my mom would leave her house was to get food or visit my grandmother. My grandmother never left the house during this time.

It was a Sunday. I had just gotten home from the hospital and finished my new "decontamination" routine where I would enter the house through the basement and put all the clothes that I was wearing in a garbage bag. Then I would clean everything I had with me (phone, keys, wallet, etc.) with a Clorox wipe, as well as everything that I touched on my way into the basement. When I got out of the shower, my mom called me and told me she was at my grandmother's house, and she was calling an ambulance because my grandmother was weak, confused, and had a fever. I knew what this meant: COVID. In late March, most patients in the emergency department had COVID. On one clinical shift during that time, 95 percent of the patients I saw had COVID.

After getting off the phone with my mother, I put scrubs back on and drove back to the hospital. My grandmother was in the emergency department. I now had two family members admitted to my hospital with COVID: my uncle and my grandmother (who was also my uncle's mother). I was able to speak to her for a while and she said she was feeling okay. She was in good spirits, and in typical "Grandma Josie" fashion, she was more concerned with asking me about how my wife and children were doing as opposed to being concerned about her own health.

Since I was the only family member that could see them,

I would go to the hospital early in the morning before work to visit them, then I would try to see them at some point during the day and once more before I went home at night. I did this routine for the next week. Initially, I did not tell my uncle that his mother was admitted to the hospital with COVID because he was still very sick at the time, and we did not want to add any extra stress to his body.

Meanwhile, my grandmother was requiring high amounts of oxygen and was extremely weak. I knew that she was facing an uphill battle and there was a high probability that she would never be able to leave the hospital. Right before my uncle was discharged, I was able to arrange for one of the nurse managers to take my uncle in a wheelchair up to visit his mother and give him a chance to see her—potentially for the last time.

Around the time my uncle was getting ready to be discharged from the hospital, my mother started having high fevers and extreme fatigue. It was obvious that she had COVID, but she was managing at home. After nine days of persistent symptoms, she was getting nervous because of everything she was hearing on the news and didn't know if she would need to be hospitalized based on her age. I was unable to see her at the time because of my work schedule, so I asked her to come to the emergency department to be evaluated. Her pulse oximetry was in the low nineties and her chest x-ray revealed classic COVID findings. Thankfully, she did not need to be admitted. I was relieved that I would not have three family members in the hospital at the same time.

In early April, a few days prior to my mom coming to the

emergency department, I received a call from the Executive Director of the hospital asking me if I would be interested in helping set up an auxiliary field hospital/facility solely for COVID patients and if I would serve as the Medical Director. At the time, I knew it was a great opportunity, and given what I was currently going through, it just felt right. I was now truly "all in" on COVID in my professional and personal life. Along with a few other colleagues, in collaboration with the State of New York and the National Guard, our leadership team of about five people set up a "hospital" in five days. We accepted our first patient on the sixth day.

Three days into the start of this project, one of my closest friends at work—who also happened to be part of the leadership team for the new hospital—sent me a message saying he had a high fever and fatigue. We knew he had COVID. My boss called me at 9 p.m. that night and told me he got us both a hotel room so we could isolate and potentially not expose our family members.

I told my wife what happened, packed my bags, and immediately left the house. My children were young (three and six at the time) and were already sleeping, so I was unable to say goodbye to them. Prior to this (ever since my uncle had been hospitalized), I had already made the decision to sleep in a different room in my house and try to avoid any contact with my children or my wife. This was by far the worst part of this experience. To see my young children and not be able to hug or kiss them because of a virus that they were too young to understand was awful.

Two days after my mom was discharged, my sister called me to tell me that she was worried about my father. I called him to see how he was doing, and he too was having similar symptoms as my mom. I already knew he had mild symptoms for a few days, but he would always minimize his symptoms. His pulse oximetry at home was in the low nineties and he was having persistent fevers. He had extreme fatigue and didn't eat much for three days, so I asked him to come to the hospital to be evaluated.

My mom, who was now recovering from COVID, drove my dad to the hospital and waited alone in the parking lot to hear whether he would be released or admitted. He was seen in the emergency department by one of my fellow attendings, who I also trained with in residency and have known for many years. We both decided that the best course of action would be to admit him to the hospital.

At this point, my uncle thankfully had already been discharged and sent home, but my grandmother was still in the hospital. My routine every day this week was the exact same: wake up early around 5 a.m., go for a run, then go to the main hospital. There, in full PPE, I would go visit my grandmother and then my father, then I would get in my car and go to the new COVID hospital for the entire day. At the end of the day, I would go back to the main hospital and visit my grandmother and father one last time, drive back to the hotel, and repeat the process the next morning.

Eventually, my grandmother started to decline and require higher amounts of oxygen. Due to the visitation policies, no one from our very large family was able to visit her in the hospital, so this responsibility fell on my shoulders. I would contact my family daily in group messages to provide updates. During this period, I was being pulled in so many directions at the same time (work, my grandmother, my father, my mother, my family). When I would leave the hospital at night, I would feel guilty that I was leaving, and I constantly had feelings that I was letting my entire family down. These were the hardest days of my life.

Late on a Friday night, I was doing my usual routine of seeing my dad and grandmother prior to going back to the hotel. I went into my grandmother's room, and I had a bad feeling. Her mental status had been worsening over the past few days and she was having difficulty communicating. I called my wife on the way to the hotel and told her I didn't think she would make it through the night.

The next morning, I got a text message from my sister that my grandmother had passed away. She died alone. Constant questions of whether or not I could have fixed this flooded my mind. *Could I have done more to help her? Should I have spent more time with her in the hospital?*

The wake and funeral service for my grandmother was surreal. Everyone was wearing masks, distanced from one another. We were only allowed to have six to eight people at the grave site while everyone else watched from the street behind the cemetery's fence—far different from the typical Italian funeral that our family is accustomed to. This was not the way we wanted to say goodbye to the matriarch of our family.

My father was unable to attend the service because he was still hospitalized, and gradually started to require more supplemental oxygen. Every time I opened the door to his room, I was nervous. I had no idea what I was going to see on the other side, which is a feeling that I would not wish on anybody.

On Easter Sunday, I decided to go back home after seeing my father in the hospital. He seemed to be doing okay that morning, so I was optimistic and hopeful, but later that day he texted me saying that they put him on a "mask" to give him more oxygen. I called the doctor who was taking care of him, and I was told he now required a non-rebreather, but his oxygen saturations were great. Later, I spoke to my dad, and he seemed okay, so I told him I would see him in the morning. However, his laboratory markers were concerning and indicative of severe COVID. He was upgraded to the ICU overnight because he was at high risk for deterioration.

The next morning when I saw my father, he was on the non-rebreather with an oxygen saturation in the eighties. At this point, I thought to myself that my father may not make it through this illness. Everything seemed to be pitted against me. A few weeks prior to this when my uncle was in the ICU, my father sent me a text message with all his bank account information just in case he got the virus and didn't make it.

Fast forward to when he was on the verge of being placed on a ventilator. I spoke to the intensivist who felt he was a good candidate for high-flow nasal cannula oxygen and did not need a ventilator at that time. He was moved to a different room in the ICU. Ironically, he was in the same exact room that my uncle was in two weeks prior, being taken care of by the exact same intensivist. It was a nightmare.

Luckily, this is where the bad story ends. My father was one of the lucky ones and was able to stay on high flow nasal oxygen for approximately one week and avoid being on a ventilator. His labs and his oxygen levels started to improve. He started to eat again. He lost approximately forty pounds while he was hospitalized. Eventually, he was transferred to the new COVID hospital where I was working, and I was able to see him throughout the day without having to go back and forth from hospital to hospital. Soon, after making great progress, he was discharged on oxygen and made a full recovery after being hospitalized for approximately one month.

As I reflect on what I went through, I realize now that I was not able to truly process what was going on, likely out of survival. I just put my head down and did what I felt like I had to do. The hardest part of the entire process was the overwhelming amount of isolation that accompanied this pandemic.

It all still haunts me: the thought of my grandmother being alone and dying alone in the hospital; having to watch my uncle get intubated alone without his wife and children at his bedside; my mother alone at home while my father was in the ICU, getting the call that her mother died alone in the hospital. The amount of pain and stress my mother had to endure is unfathomable. She had already been through so much during COVID, and now her mother was unexpectedly taken from her. She still has not had the chance to grieve appropriately.

Finally, I cannot imagine how hard it was for my wife to be home by herself with our children, constantly worrying about what was happening. She was beyond supportive, and I would never have been able to make it through this experience without her. She was my rock and a source of unconditional love and support. I was able to focus on work and my sick family members, while she took care of literally everything else. She is tougher than I will ever be.

The pandemic emphasized to me the importance of perspective, resiliency, and family support. This experience has forever changed me not only as a physician, but also as father, husband, and son. I try to reflect on the positive things, and am inspired by what my colleagues were able to accomplish during such a difficult time. My only hope is that the healthcare field continues to learn from COVID and continues to improve moving forward.

MY FIRST TRUE SAVE: THE MEANING OF OCTOBER 25TH

Dr. William Caputo

I was the first person in my family to ever become a doctor. My parents sacrificed a lot to raise my siblings and I because they wanted to give us an opportunity for a better life. This is particularly true of my mother.

My mother came to the United States from Colombia as a teenager to live with her older sister and pave her own way in America. She had to learn English, go to high school, work, and support herself. Yet, she still never let anything stop her. She made it to college on her own and started her own successful business in freight forwarding. Whatever we needed growing up, my mother would hustle and make it happen. Like my mother, I had to navigate unfamiliar waters in my pursuit of medicine.

I knew that if I could be half the person my mother was that I would be successful in life. Anything I would do would be simple compared to what she had to endure. I always wanted to make her proud and dreamed of buying her a fancy car once I could afford one.

My dreams started to become a reality when I was accepted to medical school at SUNY Downstate and things seemed to be going according to plan. Until, one day, my mother told me that she had back pain. I was finishing my second year, but wasn't educated with clinical knowledge; what I knew was mostly from my textbooks. I asked one of my teachers how I could help her and was relieved to learn that most back pain was not serious. My teacher recommended that we give it some time and make sure my mother was going to see her doctor.

On the other hand, I knew my mother was not a complainer, so it worried me when she kept bringing it up. My mother was truly the one person I could not live without, so I wanted to make sure she was healthy. Given what my teacher had told me—and that my mother worked out all the time, ate healthy, and was strict about her weight—I had no reason to believe it was anything serious. She rested for a week and said that she felt better. As a precautionary measure, she planned a visit to her doctor. All of her blood work came back normal, so I was relieved.

Shortly thereafter, the rest of my family went on vacation to Mexico. I was just starting my third year of medical school and my clinical rotations, so my schedule wasn't flexible at the time and I personally could not join my family. On one particular day of the trip, my mother had another episode of severe back pain that sidelined her. When she returned, she had insurance approval and scheduled an MRI of her lower back.

However, my mother never made it to her MRI. My brother called me days later while I was on rounds and told me they rushed my mom to Staten Island University Hospital, and she was acting erratically. My senior resident saw the panic in my eyes and told me I could leave, so I raced over to the hospital where she was admitted.

My mother had had a stroke. Her platelet count was also extremely low, and the doctors weren't sure why. After days of sleeping in the hospital, we found out that my mother had metastatic cancer that was so aggressive they couldn't even pinpoint where it started. The cancer had already invaded her bones and was all over her body, past the point where chemotherapy would help or prolong her life. There wasn't much the doctors could do, so they simply recommended making her comfortable.

My mother is the strongest person I have ever known, and she went from working out to her death bed within days. The day before she died was my younger sister's birthday, and it felt like my mother was barely holding on to make it through the day. We made her DNR/DNI and she passed away on October 25th, 2007, while I was holding her hand with my family. To this day, there is an emptiness in my life. The glue that held my family together was gone.

My anger turned into fuel to drive myself and make my mother proud. I dedicated my life to becoming the best and most compassionate doctor I could be. Throughout my residency, I tried to put into practice everything I learned from my mother. I wanted to be the doctor that went the extra mile and was never too good to perform a task. I felt at home in the emergency department. I graduated my program as a Chief Resident and was hired as an attending physician back home on Staten Island.

A lesson my mother taught me was that you can either run away from your problems or run toward and address them. After what I had gone through, it would have been easier to never step foot in Staten Island University Hospital again, but that is not how I was brought up. My goal was to bring the best care I could possibly bring to my hometown and home hospital.

On my first day working on October 25th as an attending doctor, I drove into the hospital with tears running down my face. This is the one day of the year that I don't look forward to more than any other. Despite this being an upsetting and painful car ride, at the same time, I could feel my mom's presence with me. I've always constantly had her voice in my head giving me guidance and peace.

My clinical shift that day started like any other would. I received my sign-outs from the overnight shift and got to work. I noticed I was making an extra effort to connect to all my patients and families that day. More and more patients came in and it quickly became a busy day, but it was all bread-and-butter visits and work-ups—until a thirty-two-year-old female was admitted with abdominal pain.

MY FIRST TRUE SAVE

I immediately met her bedside with the Triage nurse and my instincts immediately told me she was very sick. She was pale and writhing in pain and could only mutter that she was good friends with the head nurse of the emergency department. The first time we tried to check her blood pressure the results were inconclusive, which is concerning because she may have had severely low blood pressure. The beeping from her heart monitor sounded way too fast to be from an adult. I immediately placed a large bore IV catheter to administer medications and fluids, and moved the ultrasound machine to the patient's bedside. Within two minutes, I diagnosed that she had a belly full of blood and was at risk of bleeding to death in front of my eyes. For a woman of childbearing age, this is a ruptured ectopic pregnancy until proven otherwise. A ruptured ectopic pregnancy is one unfortunate diagnosis that continues to claim many young women every year.

My emergency medicine training kicked into full gear. There was no time to wait for a pregnancy test or for blood work to result. I drew some extra blood when I placed her IV—a shortcut I learned from one of my favorite attendings—and used it on a bedside pregnancy test. Two lines immediately showed up; it was positive. Until blood was ready, we had to start an intravenous fluid as quickly as possible to restore volume and hopefully get a blood pressure reading.

Now that the diagnosis was made, I needed to keep my patient alive and get her to the operating room STAT for emergency surgery. This was the moment that makes the emergency department and the people who work there as great as they are. There were so many things that had to happen from this point on to ensure the patient's safety. I called to the charting room and to the other nursing staff for help.

"All Hands Team to Bed 4" our clerk immediately called out. Leadership had established an overhead call for moments like this, and it meant that everyone working should immediately come to the room to help.

I knew everything that we needed—OB-GYN STAT, the operating room ready, medications, blood products. We also had to get consent for blood transfusion and emergency surgery. Separately, we needed to make sure the patient and her family knew what was going on and what the plan was. There were at least twenty steps that needed to be done—quickly—to help save this person's life.

My patient was suffering from hypovolemic shock due to blood loss. The only way to fix this is to stop the bleeding and replace the blood that the patient lost. I immediately placed a sixteen-gauge IV in the patient's other arm, which is the best way to resuscitate someone that needs blood or fluid. When you are bleeding so much, your veins are flat, so an IV of this size can sometimes be hard to place. With precision, I successfully threaded this catheter into her vein so that intravenous calcium and other blood products like platelets and fresh frozen plasma could be administered to restore the blood components the patient was exsanguinating.

We checked the patient's vital signs every two to three minutes. The primary nurse did not leave her bedside. She was the eyes and ears for the patient and updated the team with any changes in status.

Meanwhile, one of the residents ran like a track star to the Blood Bank to get numerous units of blood for immediate transfusion. Simultaneously, the "Level I" infuser, which could infuse warmed blood into someone, needed to be primed and troubleshot to help transfuse the blood products, so the charge nurse put their other duties on pause and jumped right on this. The hum of this machine working was music to my ears. Another nurse procured all the medicine we needed, while the other primed and prepped the blood tubing for infusion. Before I could turn around, the consent forms were handed to me and were filled out by one of our great PAs. Our clerk had also gotten the OB-GYN attending on the phone and transferred the call to my portable Spectra. The other emergency department attending helped place all her orders and spoke with the Operating Room staff.

The patient had been here for less than fifteen minutes.

We didn't even have a formal pregnancy test yet or blood work results, let alone an ultrasound from Radiology. When I told the consulting doctor the patient's brief story, that I was ultrasound trained, and that she had a positive FAST exam with blood in her abdomen, I was able to convince the OB-GYN attending that I had made the correct diagnosis and recruited an extremely valuable member to my team. She informed us that she was rushing in and to have the operating room ready.

Two units of blood went in rapid fire, and we finally got a detectable blood pressure. It was 80/50, which is still extremely low, but is a big step up from being too low to measure. As a few more minutes went by and we got into the third and fourth unit, her blood pressure continued to rise, and her heart rate was improving. I couldn't help but think that if we were delayed by even a few more minutes that this patient would have flatlined, and we would have been doing chest compressions to try and revive her heart.

The nursing staff assisted me in placing the patient on a portable monitor, and we then rushed toward the elevator to deliver her to the operating room. It was up to our OB-GYN colleague to take over and finish saving her life. Another great thing about emergency medicine is that we know when help is needed and what limitations we have. The patient was delivered safely to the OR with better vital signs, and it wouldn't be long before we knew the outcome of the case.

Back down in the emergency department, her room was empty, but all the equipment, empty blood products, and other medication bags were proof of our efforts. We debriefed with the team for a few minutes to go over the case and address any questions in the room since there wasn't much time to discuss what was happening in the moment.

My adrenaline was still coursing through my veins, and I could not wait to hear about her outcome from the operating room. I knew I did the best I could, but at this point, it was out of my hands. I had lost people previously and knew if I heard an overhead announcement of "Code Blue to the operating room," which is when someone's heart stops in our hospital, that our chances were minimal.

Instead of an overhead announcement, the emergency department phone rang. The OB-GYN attending was ecstatic on the phone and told me that the patient was saved in surgery. She had well over two liters of blood in her abdomen, but it was now controlled, and we were in the clear. I hung up the phone and shared the great news with the rest of the team. Excitement and relief filled the department.

In a true storybook ending, we learned of the outcome at the exact moment that the patient's husband got back to the emergency room, this time with their son, whom he had just rushed to pick up from school. I will never forget them turning the corner and walking toward us and heading to Room 4.

Before the husband could even speak, their seven-year-old son asked me: "Doctor, is my mom OK?" Looking into this young child's innocent eyes, it would've broken me if I had to give them bad news. I happily responded to this young boy's question by saying that everything was going to work out fine and not to worry at all. I don't think he'll ever know how close he came to losing his mother on that day. I still haven't gotten over the loss of my mom, and I was twenty-five years old at the time.

Seeing and updating the family made our celebration in the emergency department that much more meaningful. It was our accomplishment and our great save. Although I was the attending on the case, everyone in the emergency department chipped in to make this happen. Moments like this make our job all worth it; they make you want to be better for the next case.

Reflecting on this experience, this had been the encounter I was training for my whole career. My mother instilled in me to never settle and always be the best I can be. Those hundreds of hours of bedside ultrasound and my advanced ultrasound degree made me ready for this moment. The thousands of IVs I pushed myself to continue to place also were extremely useful. When seconds mattered, I was there when I needed to be and did not let this patient down. I truly felt a sense that I was supposed to be there in that particular moment to help save this woman's life.

To this day, you will catch me working on October 25th. Almost year in and year out, I come across a case that reminds me of why I am supposed to be working on this day. I do it for my mom and I hope to continue to make her proud.

THE NEAR-DEATH EXPERIENCES

DR. JAMES F. KENNY SR.

Carpe diem quam minimum credula postero. Seize the day, trusting as little as possible in the next one.

It was a sultry July morning. It was a Friday, and I had taken the day off. As per my morning routine, I was sitting in my kitchen having a bowl of Cheerios while reading the paper. I had the sliding glass door open, listening to the southern Staten Island sounds of summer: mockingbirds singing and lawn mowers wailing.

For me, it was a typical summer day; I had not showered or shaved yet in anticipation of running later in the morning. My hair looked like it was combed with a firecracker. I was wearing an old torn T-shirt. The front of the shirt was an ad for Arrogant Bastard Ale; the back of the shirt read, "You are not worthy." My ensemble was completed with my typical green Cabela shorts that I would wear for the rest of the summer along with my well-broken-in moose skin moccasins.

I was alone in the house except for my daughter, Megan,

who was sleeping soundly upstairs. She was recuperating from her first year of college by sleeping until the crack of noon daily. She would then "seize the day" by watching alternating reruns of *Ghostbusters I* and *II*.

I suddenly heard a piercing scream from a woman who lived behind my next-door neighbor. I had never seen or met these people who lived in that house. My backyard is lined by twelve-foot juniper trees, so unfortunately, I could not see what the source of the commotion was. I started shouting and asking if anybody needed help, but instead, I just heard the screaming over and over again. Somewhere between the screams and yelling I heard, "Baby! . . . Pool!"

I immediately ran to the bottom of the stairs, and I screamed to Megan to get up. Three times I shouted, "Get up, go to the backyard, and do whatever I say!" I grabbed the keys to my car, and I drove around the corner as fast as I could. I parked in the middle of the street in front of the screaming neighbor's house.

I later found out that the house with all the screaming was owned by a retired couple who were grandparents; they were watching their grandson who was about fourteen months old. Grandma must have had the child-safe slider open when the phone rang. She did not realize her grandson had wandered into the backyard and went into the pool. After an unknown amount of time, she went outside and found the toddler floating motionlessly, and that was when the screaming started.

I had arrived just behind the twenty-something-year-old

son of my neighbor. We immediately extracted the child from the pool. His body was strikingly white, like snow.

He was not breathing, and had no pulse.

The child was in cardiac arrest.

I asked my fellow rescuer if he knew how to do CPR; he verified he most certainly did and had just finished EMT training a few weeks ago! He started doing chest compressions while I started doing mouth-to-mouth ventilation. After what seemed like an eternity (even though it was probably just a couple of minutes), I heard the sound of sirens. It felt like the cavalry was coming. An ambulance and a fire truck pulled up to the house, and the medics made their way into the backyard. The medics wore Staten Island University Hospital (SIUH) patches on their uniforms. I asked them, "Are you paramedics or EMTs?" and they identified themselves as such.

In my judgment, this baby's best chance was to be intubated as soon as possible, and to receive advanced resuscitative measures; the BLS (Basic Life Support) ambulance would not have the required equipment or medications available. I picked up the baby, ran to the street with the medics behind me, and placed the baby onto the stretcher in the back of the ambulance. With no regard to the fact that I probably outwardly appeared like a hungover charter boat captain, I started directing the medics to do chest compressions, "No, faster! Faster! It's a baby!"

I put an oral airway into the toddler's mouth, and I ordered the EMT to start bag-valve-mouth ventilations.

There was a firefighter at the scene who knew how to drive the ambulance, so I directed him to get behind the wheel and start driving toward the hospital. Within a few seconds, we were on our way with sirens blasting.

The closest hospital is SIUH/South: the emergency department where I had been working for over twenty years at the time. We were quickly rolling down Hylan Boulevard when I heard chatter on the radio. The paramedic ambulance—"23 Willie"—was directing the EMTs to pull over and meet them on Page Avenue which is approximately two miles from the hospital. Their plan was to take over care of the child from the EMTs.

I shouted at the driver, "Bypass 23 Willie! I say again: bypass 23 Willie! Go directly to Hospital 59!"

"Hospital 59" is the EMS designation for SIUH/South.

"Make notification to Hospital 59. Stand by for incoming critical pediatric. 1½-year-old male. CPR in progress. Victim of drowning. Will require intubation. ETA two minutes. Make notification now!"

The medics made the notification as I requested. We were still about a minute away from the ED when one of the medics said, "You really seem to know what you are talking about . . . are you an EMT or something?"

I yelled, "No, I am Jim Kenny . . . I am one of your medical directors!" The crew's eyes widened, and their jaws slacked as they realized who this beach bum barking orders at them was. Although I had interacted with the crew for many years, they did not recognize me without my traditional scrubs and white coat. In spite of that, they followed my orders to the letter. It just goes to show it is sometimes more important how you deliver a message than who the messenger is.

As we were backing up to the entrance of the emergency department, I picked up the baby off the stretcher and opened the ambulance door while it was still moving. I leapt out and ran to the resuscitation bay where the emergency department team was awaiting the child. The team continued CPR and placed a cardiac monitor on the child.

Interestingly, while the child still had no pulse, he had cardiac electrical activity at a rate of about ten complexes per minute. Dr. Pilat was the attending on duty. She promptly intubated the child while I shot an intraosseous device into the child's shin bone so we could immediately deliver resuscitative medications. After one or two minutes, following positive pressure ventilation via the endotracheal tube and an intraosseous dose of epinephrine, he started getting a pulse back, his heart rate picked up, and he had a measurable blood pressure. For the first time, I said to myself, *Oh, my God! This child just might make it!*

As the child continued to improve, I started to put the whole scenario together in my head. The child must have experienced what is known as the "diving reflex," which almost all mammals have the capacity to experience. Nerve receptors on the chest wall are responsible for this phenomenon. When these nerve receptors sense pressure and/or cold water, they send the signal to the heart to slow down. In addition, the reflex causes the arteries to the muscles, the gut, and the kidneys to constrict. Essentially, all the blood is confined to a tight little circulation between the heart and the brain. As a result, little oxygen is consumed elsewhere in the body for an extended period of time. This diving reflex is well-developed in marine mammals, which is why when dolphins and whales breach, they hit their chest on cold water, intentionally initiating the diving reflex. Once the diving reflex starts, marine mammals can stay under water for a pretty long time. The diving reflex is far less developed in humans. Children tend to experience a significantly more exaggerated diving reflex than adults. This is why there are numerous reports of young children being resuscitated after drowning in cold water after an extended period of time.

This young boy walked out of the kitchen, fell into the pool, and hit his chest square onto the surface of a cold-water pool. This triggered the diving reflex. Although his heart was not beating, he was not using a lot of oxygen. Following his rescue from the pool, he received professional level CPR and within ten minutes of the initiation of CPR, he was getting advanced and expert care in the emergency department of SIUH/South.

As soon the child started to stabilize, I backed away from further patient care. I witnessed some action going on in the waiting room. Apparently, the grandmother was so despondent that she tried to grab the handgun out of a cop's holster because she wanted to kill herself. The emergency department staff registered her as a patient and gave her something to calm her down.

THE NEAR-DEATH EXPERIENCES

At SIUH/South, there is no inpatient pediatric unit. Any pediatric patient that requires admission must be transferred to SIUH/North. It wasn't long before the paramedic transfer ambulance showed up, and the paramedics prepared the child for the ambulance ride to the North Site PICU. At that time, I approached the grandfather to introduce myself. I gave him my card with my cell phone number, and I explained that if he had any problems or communication difficulties at the North Site, I could serve as a resource to him and his family. I also wrote my home address on the card and encouraged him to knock on my door at any time if he had any problems or he wanted to talk.

Grandpa recounted, "Hey, doc, you do not have to write your home address on the card. Everybody in the neighborhood knows you and where you live. You are the doctor who plays basketball and wiffle ball in front of your house and runs a pool party with your kids every day of the summer." I was pretty happy that my neighbors thought of me that way. As a doctor, your career can sometimes overwhelm other aspects of your life. Extracting time from your family life seems to be the easiest way to compensate for most of the people in my profession, and sometimes those closest to you can suffer. If I can be remembered as the guy who played ball with his kids when they were growing up, that is a great legacy as far as I am concerned.

This kid actually recovered amazingly well. Within a few days, thanks to daily miracles by Dr. Chan and the PICU staff, he was extubated. He spent about three weeks at the

North Site, and then he was transferred to a rehabilitation hospital in New Jersey. I checked up on him while he was in the hospital several times, but after he was discharged, I did not hear from the family for a while. The next time I saw him was Halloween. On that day, some four months later, he was able to go trick-or-treating at my house. I was astonished he was able to walk on his own, and that he was able to talk.

Seeing that little boy smiling on my front porch reminded me why I chose this profession.

After that Halloween, I did not receive much follow-up regarding our little patient until 2022. One day, I went to the lab supervisor's office to discuss some administrative matters. After we finished our discussion, she asked out of the blue, "What year did you save a child from drowning in the pool?" I told her 2010. She proceeded to show me a video on her cell phone of a team of twelve-year-old boys playing in an organized full-court basketball game. One of the boys definitely had strong dribbling ability and a decent outside shot for a boy that age. To my surprise, she identified that talented young basketball player as the young boy we saved from drowning twelve years ago. I had a big smile on my face for the rest of the week!

As a sidebar, I also learned a valuable life lesson from my experience caring for this child. My brother Mike was a police detective for NYPD, and he used to say in his professional experience "the worst witness is an eyewitness." He used to say this because in the eyes of the law, the testimony of an eyewitness is always given considerable weight. Mike would explain that any experienced police detective knows that the eyewitness' memory can quickly and dramatically be altered by their emotions and personal biases and can continue to morph even more as time passes after the original incident. He pointed out that your mind tries to reconstruct what happened and as you start telling people the story, the story sometimes becomes the memory, and it can be a little— or a lot—different from what actually happened.

I recall a couple of days after this child was in the hospital, I went around the block to see the grandparents, make sure the hospital staff was communicating effectively to the family, and see if they needed any help or explanations. The grandfather refused, saying that I had already done enough. He then added that "until the day he died," he would "never forget" how "I leapt over the fence" from the house on my street into his backyard and dove in the pool and plucked out his grandson and started CPR. He told the story with such emotion and drama, and although that is not the way it happened, who am I to deprive him of an emotionally charged memory? Anyway, it seemed to be a much more exciting story than me driving around block. . . .

It is funny how the story gained a life of its own because so many other people repeated it. The story actually became "fact." Some ten years later after the incident, I saw one of the doctors who took care of the boy while he was in the PICU. I saw this doctor as a patient in the ER. His wife was at his bedside; he introduced me to his wife as the "doctor who jumped over a fence" and saved the kid from drowning in a pool.

THE EMERGENCY DIARIES

For many years after this incident, I would occasionally wonder what that boy remembered during those ten or fifteen minutes that he was in cardiac arrest it. For me, it is a fascinating phenomenon that some emergency physicians have experienced up close after they resuscitated somebody and then heard the stories of what the patient remembered.

I have witnessed a few of these incidents in my career. Perhaps one of the most vivid was that of a gentleman who was complaining of chest pain. I was alone with him at his bedside in the trauma room of SIUH/South peering down at a very concerning EKG: this guy was having an acute STEMI (a.k.a. heart attack). I was getting some additional history and started to examine him when, suddenly, he went into "v fib" cardiac arrest. Right away, I yelled for help. The emergency department tech was the first to arrive, and he started doing CPR. The nurses came into the room to give us a hand. I intubated the patient right away. His veins were bad, so I put an IV in his neck to administer ACLS meds. After the second round of epinephrine—and at least five minutes of CPR—we got him back. We shocked him four times before we got a pulse. Within an hour of the resuscitation, he was totally alert and trying to pull the tube out, so I decided to extubate him. After we stabilized him, and he was about to go to the CCU (Coronary Care Unit), I asked him if he remembered anything. He said, "I most certainly do remember . . . I remember you were talking to me when all of a sudden everything became dark. I seemed to slip out of the darkness, and I found myself floating above my body in the emergency room. I remember there was a blond-haired guy doing chest compressions: he was on the left side of the bed. You were on the right side of the bed, and you were trying to put something in my neck." I was amazed that he was able to describe the two nurses that also assisted in his resuscitation, including their hair color and where they were standing relative to his stretcher.

He continued his story. "After a short while, I was no longer floating above my body. Instead, I found myself in the back of a large church. In the front of the church, there was an altar with a very bright stained-glass window over it. I found myself walking down the center aisle of the church. In the pews, there were people I recognized as long-since dead relatives. I got to the altar where my father was waiting for me. Again, my father had died many years ago. He handed me a small glass. . . . I took a sniff from the glass, and it smelled like a strong brandy. I brought the glass to my lips, and I was about to take a sip, but then I stopped—and I handed the glass back to my father. Suddenly, I found myself back in my body."

I was always impressed by the vividness of his story. My takeaway: Since there was no mention of a tab, there may be an open bar in heaven.

They say death is the "undiscovered country." We are taught to fear this inevitable trek into *terra incognita* as young children. My experience as an emergency physician forces the dead and the dying into the front row of my clinical shifts on a daily basis. I have come to realize how we face death is almost as important as we face life. The near-death experiences of my patients give me a degree of solace that death is not an end, and the people closest to me are waiting for me, and I will be waiting for the ones who come after me.

This makes me less afraid.

PEDIATRIC DEATH

Dr. Eric S. Levy

I awoke to the usual sound of my alarm clock blaring from my nightstand. My eyes opened slowly as I checked the clock— 4:30 A.M. I remember setting the alarm the night before as I was scrolling through my phone in bed much later than I should have been, blissfully ignorant of the true pain I would feel when the time to wake up would finally arrive. I heard the familiar sound of my twenty-month-old daughter crying as my wife consoled her. It had been the usual night of sleep for my beloved little princess—sleeping until around 3 a.m., with only broken sleep thereafter. I love her and my son with all my heart, and yet sometimes I wonder how much more rested I would be if they actually slept.

I took my time slowly making my way to the shower, and then downstairs to make myself breakfast as I heard the soothing sound of my daughter's calm breathing through the baby monitor. I sighed in relief, as now I knew my wife would be able to rest for at least a little longer. I made my coffee and then made my way to my car as the familiar heated leather seats greeted me. It was a particularly chilly morning, and the feeling of heat combined with sipping my hot coffee soothed my mind.

Throughout my medical training to this point, I felt invincible. I had seen a tremendous number of patients of all backgrounds and ages and stabilized the sickest of the sick. I felt confident despite my expected apprehension of the responsibility one carries as an attending.

On the drive to the hospital, my mind blurred to what I consider to be a landmark case in my very young career thus far.

*   *   *

During one of my last residency shifts, we received an EMS call for a fifty-year-old male, hypotensive and vomiting blood, about ten minutes away. I went through my usual routine of preparing the trauma bay, having all the necessary airway equipment ready and preparing emergency release blood at bedside ready for transfusion. My attending at the time joined me in the room, nodding to me as if to say it was my show to run.

The patient arrived awake and surprisingly in good spirits. He looked very pale and fragile, but his eyes seemed kind and youthful. He had been driving home with his wife after dinner, at which time he felt suddenly nauseous and pulled to the side of the road to vomit, which he noted to be dark and bloody, so his wife called 911. He denied any medical history and was never on any medications. He had crusted blood on his lips, but was not actively vomiting during my exam. His vital signs were surprisingly stable on arrival, and he was mentating appropriately. As I was leaving to enter my orders for blood work, he pulled me aside and leaned in close.

"I'm in your hands, doc," he said with a lighthearted smile. "Today's not my day to die."

I smiled back with a nod as I entered my orders. I had seen so many of these kinds of cases, and learned never to trust the stability of a gastrointestinal bleed.

As soon as I had entered my orders, the nurse called me back to the trauma bay as the patient began vomiting blood and was becoming lethargic. My attending and I rushed to the scene, revealing the patient covered in dark blood, breathing heavily, only semiconscious, with his blood pressure dropping. I acted quickly and started transfusing the emergency release blood through a rapid infuser, and activated the mass transfusion protocol, which is a hospital-wide notification necessary to obtain a large amount of blood products emergently. With the blood running rapidly, the patient's blood pressure improved, but he remained lethargic, and his oxygen level began to slowly decline. I knew I did not have much time, as he likely aspirated the blood, and without intubation, he would continue to decline and likely go into cardiac arrest. I prepared for intubation with my attending at bedside, who I knew would no longer be there as backup once I graduated in a few short weeks.

As the medications were pushed to sedate and paralyze the patient prior to intubation, I entered the blade into his mouth and began my search for his vocal cords. During my residency and training, I had intubated hundreds of patients prior to this, yet this particular intubation still to this day causes my heart to skip a beat.

As soon as I opened his mouth, a tremendous amount of blood exploded onto my shielded face, covering me and all of the ED personnel nearby at the head of the bed. As if by sheer instinct alone, I reached for the suction and began suctioning as much as I could. However, it seemed for every clump of blood I would suction, ten times that amount would reappear in the mouth. I began to internally panic as I glanced up at the patient's monitor—his oxygen saturation had begun to decline to the eighties, and I knew there wasn't much time.

Another wave of blood projected from his mouth onto my face shield as I continued to search the back of his mouth. We had video laryngoscopy at my residency, which shows the whole picture of the back of the patient's throat on a screen for the room to see, but unfortunately for this intubation, the blood would make this impossible due to the camera being blocked, and therefore we had to resort to direct visualization of his vocal cords with a plain intubation blade. As I frantically searched the back of his mouth, I could hear the charge nurse beside me whispering to me in support, as she could sense my fear.

"Come on, Levy, you got this."

As if by some miracle, I saw a glimpse of the familiar white rim of his vocal cords under a rather large epiglottis covered in dark blood. It was now or never. I quickly maneuvered the tube down the back of his mouth and successfully into his vocal cords, down his trachea. A sigh of relief silenced the room as the patient's oxygen level began to improve with manual ventilation.

The patient ultimately survived after we transfused unit after unit of blood products, and Gastroenterology performed an emergent endoscopy in the ER to stop the bleeding. It was one of the most difficult intubations of my young career, and despite my emotions, I had persevered and saved the patient's life. It was after this case that I truly felt ready to begin my journey as an attending physician.

* * *

My mind snapped back to the present as I pulled into a parking space near the hospital. A pediatric ER shift is arguably my least favorite. My confidence always seems to hit an abrupt end when it comes to the pediatric population. Children are wonderful and truly a gift to humankind, but when they are sick, the weight of the world can be on their doctors' shoulders. I absolutely dread my pediatric shifts. While it typically involves a bunch of Motrin and what we call "TLC," or "tender loving care," for both the patients and their parents, for their mostly non-emergent runny noses, there is always that potential catastrophe lurking in the shadows—a truly sick or even dying pediatric patient ready to make even the most experienced doctors quiver to the bone.

"Let's do this," I mumbled to myself as I reached for my stethoscope and ID badge.

I looked in the rearview mirror one last time before exiting my car, amicably nodding at various coworkers as I headed directly to the pediatric area. Greeting me was the familiar face of one of my favorite senior residents, with whom I have worked many unforgettable shifts and whom I fully trust to assist me to the fullest extent, even during the most taxing of shifts.

The day started as it usually did in the pediatric emergency department—the usual slew of runny noses, coughs (for one day), fever (for which nothing was given by parents prior to arrival), the patient with reported "abdominal pain" that is munching on Cheetos during my evaluation. I felt almost robotic as I went room to room with the resident.

"I don't see any signs of bacterial infection, which is a good sign." I would say, "This seems more like a virus. There are a lot of viruses going around this year, it's just terrible. I feel like my kids are constantly passing things between each other! Unfortunately, antibiotics don't work for viruses, and we just have to let this thing run its course until the body kills it. Make sure to hydrate well at home, take Motrin and Tylenol for the fever, and if anything gets worse or if the fever lasts more than five straight days, come back so we can reassess."

This usually seemed to ease the minds of the clearly worried parents who had, it seemed, never seen the common cold before. It was bread-and-butter pediatric emergency medicine, and unfortunately while it remains this way a huge proportion of the time, there is always the potential of danger lurking.

It was around 11 a.m. by this point and we had cleared out the department, making rapid dispositions effortlessly and bringing my patient list down to zero for the first time since the beginning of the shift. One would think this would normally satisfy me, but today a chill in the air swept through the halls. I am not really the superstitious type, but there is an old adage in emergency medicine, and that is to never utter the word "quiet" and to never celebrate too early.

We had just finished printing the final discharge papers when we heard the familiar shrill of the red phone in the critical care area of the emergency room. Normally, this phone is reserved for paramedic call-aheads—primarily for strokes, traumas, heart attacks, cardiac arrests, and the like. A large portion of the time, these cases are adult, and during a pediatric shift, I am blissfully ignorant of such calls. Sometimes, however, it is an omen that the worst is yet to come.

My work phone buzzed in my jacket pocket. I glanced down, expecting it to be perhaps a wrong number, as I did not have any active patients, or it could have even been my colleagues on the adult section, asking if I would like to join them in a lunch order. My relative naivete rapidly faded however when I heard the cold tone of the charge nurse on the other end.

"Dr. Levy," he said, "we need you in the critical care area emergently."

I took a deep breath, as I let those words settle in my mind. I was not working a critical care shift that day. *Could the critical care attending perhaps be overwhelmed and need assistance?* This was the best-case scenario. However, I knew this was not the case.

"We have a pediatric cardiac arrest coming, about ten minutes out. Eight months old," he replied, his tone remaining cold.

"I'm on my way," I said as I hung up. My senior resident was watching me closely at this point, resting her forehead in her hands, reading my expression with utter terror in her eyes.

"There's a pediatric cardiac arrest ten minutes out," I said, my voice trailing. Cardiac arrests, at least on the adult side, do not scare me the same way they did when I was an intern in residency. My experience to this point has shown me that cardiac arrests are algorithmic, even robotic at times. A rigid set of protocols is followed depending on the cardiac rhythm the patient is in as well as the chances of achieving the coveted ROSC (or "return of spontaneous circulation"). Pediatric cardiac arrests, however, are an entirely different animal.

Without a doubt, the advanced life support algorithm for pediatrics is just as rigid and methodical as it is in adult medicine. However, it is in our human nature to allow our emotions during these cases to overcome our logic. In our logical-yet-fragile minds, the death of a ninety-year-old grandparent is sad without a doubt, but almost expected. He or she has lived ninety years on this Earth, and it is expected that by that point the human body begins to decline. When a patient is relatively young, but still considered an adult, it is tragic as well, but also expected in the appropriate context—a motor vehicle accident, a drug overdose, or even a gunshot wound. Children, however, regardless of circumstance, are never expected. There is never a clear mind in that trauma bay when a pediatric case arrives, regardless of experience level.

"I have everything ready," my resident said as I looked at her setup of the usual airway materials, including a variety of endotracheal tubes, suction, bag valve mask, and of course the intubation blade connected firmly to the video laryngoscope. The team of critical care nurses and technicians gathered in the eerily quiet room, with palpable apprehension cutting through the silence. I always hated this part. The waiting time can conjure some of the most horrific and defeatist thoughts in one's mind prior to the patient's arrival. Worst-case scenarios make their horrid way into our deepest thoughts, clouding our judgment and heightening our emotions, making us question our capabilities and skill sets we have trained so hard to perfect.

Then, the familiar beeping of the ambulance as it backed into the parking bay outside.

"They're here everyone!" I called out, as everyone hesitantly took their places. I took a deep breath as I watched the paramedics down the hallway rushing a stretcher down toward the trauma bay, one of the paramedics actively doing compressions while another was delivering breaths via the bag valve mask. It was showtime.

"Eight-month-old female in arrest," the tallest of the three paramedics announced as he helped to wheel the stretcher into the trauma bay.

"She was last seen alive by parents one hour ago prior to her nap. Reportedly, she was at a birthday celebration with family and was then put down for her nap by her mother. After one hour, her parents checked on her and she was not breathing, so 911 was called." The words barely made it out of his breathless lungs as he helped to move the patient to our ED stretcher.

"Unknown exact down time," he continued.

"We attempted intubation en route but were unsuccessful, so we bagged her on the way. She was in PEA on our arrival, but for the past five minutes or so she has been in asystole. We have been doing ongoing compressions and she has received a total of four epinephrines, no shocks."

I watched as the room slowly erupted into somewhat-organized chaos—one of our technicians immediately began doing compressions on the patient, the nursing team scrambled to attach cardiac leads to the patient to monitor her rhythm and establish intravenous access, and the respiratory therapist began delivering oxygen to the patient via a bag valve mask.

In my mind, I knew I had to stay calm. One of the things I had learned during my residency training is that no matter how chaotic or emotional a case may be, those present in the room will tend to mirror the emotion of their leader. As the attending physician, I was captain of the ship, and regardless of how scared or emotional I may be, I must at least appear calm, methodical, confident, and lead my team through this. A panicked leader will surely have panicked followers, and panic destroys efficiency in these critical situations.

I slowly went through the pediatric advanced life support algorithm in my head as compressions were ongoing. My resident began the process of intubation while I immediately called for calcium, magnesium, bicarbonate, and more epinephrine from the code cart in an attempt to get the heart to start again.

"What do you see?" I asked the resident as she was attempting to intubate.

"I—I can't see anything," she stammered. "There's too much blood."

She began suctioning as the respiratory therapist began bagging the patient again to deliver oxygen in the interim. I quickly made my way to the head of the bed and reached for the intubation blade. My mind briefly flashed back to the gastrointestinal bleed from residency as I opened the patient's tiny mouth and slid the blade inside.

I have successfully intubated many difficult airways in my relatively young career, and yet, no matter how good one's muscle memory is, the heat of the moment can have a significant weight on one's performance. As I began to look, panic began to set in—I couldn't see any landmarks. Typically, with intubation, the ultimate goal is to find the epiglottis, as this is the gatekeeper to the final destination—the vocal cords. A wall of red blocked my vision though as I frantically began searching. I glanced up at the door to the trauma bay and reminded myself of my thoughts during the gastrointestinal bleed intubation—this time, however, I was on my own. I was the end-all, and therefore failure was not an option. My mind snapped back to the present as I saw a sliver of red that appeared to be a different shade from the rest of the blood pooling in the mouth—it was a red balloon, blending almost perfectly with the blood.

"There's a balloon in the airway!" I yelled aloud as compressions were ongoing. Chills went down my spine as I envisioned what must have happened. She was at a birthday party and there must have been a balloon near or around her crib that she ingested, causing her to suffocate. I took a deep breath as I was holding back my tears. I now knew resuscitation was futile. This entire time, a balloon had been in her airway and even with paramedics trying to deliver oxygen, nothing was passing the balloon and therefore no oxygen was ever delivered.

I reached for forceps and removed the balloon, bringing the vocal cords blatantly into view. In one swift move, I maneuvered the intubation tube into the vocal cords as the respiratory therapist connected the patient to the ventilator. I clutched the balloon tightly in my gloved hand as I choked back my emotions. I glanced up at the trauma bay windowed door, through which I could see the patient's parents holding each other and crying. This piece of rubber—this single piece of cheap insignificant material had cost this patient her life.

PEDIATRIC DEATH

The rest of the resuscitation remains a blur in my mind. I remember on each subsequent pulse check, the patient remained in asystole, and ultimately, we used a bedside ultrasound to visualize the heart—no activity. There was nothing else we could do. She was gone. I called time of death, then spoke at length with the emotional parents, after which time I excused myself from the bay. There was not a single dry eye in the trauma bay. I stepped outside to collect myself, staring into the distance as my eyes watered. No matter how strong one tries to be in these situations, showing emotion is always inevitable.

I returned to the trauma bay and debriefed with my team, as is common practice. This allows us to look at the situation with hindsight, seeing what could have been done better, and how we can improve for next time. It also helps us all come to terms with the ultimate result together. I glanced at the clock—1 p.m. My shift ended at 7 p.m. One of the most difficult parts of my job is compartmentalization. We see some truly fascinating, yet terrifying things in the emergency department—things that could make amazing stories at a social gathering. And still, no matter what we see, or whom we encounter, there is always the next patient to be seen. That next patient does not know, nor care, about what you had seen that day. They care about how you can help them right now.

As part of my residency training, I have learned to compartmentalize my emotion until the end of the shift and leave it all behind. However, for the remainder of my shift, my resident and I remained in a daze. We saw another slew of runny noses and coughs, removed a splinter, splinted a broken leg, all as if we were on autopilot. There was an unspoken tension in the air amongst all of us in the ER since this tragic event, and no matter how much we tried, we could not return to normalcy. I had just discharged one of my last patients as I felt a calm hand on my shoulder. I immediately looked up to see my colleague here to relieve me, as my shift had ended. I smiled at him as I signed out my computer. It was time to go home.

My drive home flew by in an instant. My wife had put the kids to sleep by this point, but I didn't care. I immediately ran upstairs and hugged each of them tightly, sobbing into their pajama tops and waking them both up to my wife's dismay.

I love my job. I think it is the best job in the world. However, one thing I deeply fear, and yet truly extol, about this field of work is that no matter how confident one may be, it will always find a way to humble and remind that one must always stay prepared for anything we may encounter.

As emergency physicians, we cannot save everyone. However, most times we can make a genuine difference in people's lives. We see people on the worst days of their lives, and yet we are trained to be jacks of all trades, able to solve any medical problem we may face, and be the saving life-force bringing them out of an approaching darkness. I use this mentality as my motivation to continue my practice as an emergency physician. No matter how hard things may have been, I still must always remain prepared for that next patient to come through those hospital doors requiring my immediate attention.

PERSPECTIVE

DR. NIMA MAJLESI

The emergency department is a place where no one other than those of us who are built for the chaos would ever want to spend much time. Not many people can handle the unpredictability of this organized chaos. Over the years, I have learned to embrace the chaos of my work environment. Occasionally, I even thrive in it. I recall one shift, where I was managing four dying patients in our critical care area of the emergency department, when I noticed one of the neurologists staring at me. I felt her gaze as I walked (briskly) from room to room, barking orders and ensuring I was guiding the care of patients in the right direction. After I had a moment to finally take a breath, I finally looked back at her. She looked me directly in the eyes and sincerely said, "I could never do what you do."

It wasn't clear to me if she was pitying me at that moment, or if she admired my ability to practice emergency medicine. My response was a sheepish "... well, I have been trained well to do this." What I actually wanted to say was "I know you can't." It wasn't conceit that made that inner response so natural for me. Because I could easily say to her the same line (I never had any interest in being a neurologist). But I know that emergency medicine is a calling and a natural fit for many of us who choose this field.

Each year, when I visit my ophthalmologist for my eye exam, he reminds me of his days during residency. Most people don't realize that comparatively, emergency medicine is a relatively new primary specialty in the house of medicine. Years of horrendous care in emergency departments led some physicians to realize that having physicians specifically trained in this specialty was important. Before this, young doctors who had just graduated medical school that were doing residencies in other specialties (such as ophthalmology) staffed emergency departments. My ophthalmologist was one of those young physicians, who covered the emergency department right after medical school to make extra money while he was doing his residency. We call this "moonlighting."

At the time, there was no specific training required to work in an emergency department, and often it was the least-qualified physicians who could not obtain residencies in specialties such as internal medicine, surgery, and pediatrics, which frequently led to substandard care. My ophthalmologist would tell me stories of his confusion and desperation as he tried to manage multiple critically ill patients with little training and experience. He always made me feel good with words of admiration, and he was convinced it was one of the most challenging specialties in medicine.

However, in my eyes, the emergency department is a microcosm of life. Despite being well-prepared, trained, educated, and experienced, there are moments that you cannot prepare for. Unusual medical, social, and emotional situations leave a mark on your soul. My second year as an attending left me with one of my "marks."

The morning started with a sprint. A few hours into the shift, one of our very new attendings, Dr. X, called me and said her mom was heading in and might be in the waiting room already. Her mother had been complaining of chest pain and had a history of heart issues. Dr. X said she would drive in shortly, but asked if I could see her mother and let her know what I thought. If there was one benefit to working in healthcare, it was that most of us went above and beyond for each other.

As I awaited her mother's arrival, I continued to move through the patients waiting to be seen. Shortly thereafter, I received a phone call from the critical care area to come see an unstable patient. I walked into the trauma bay to find a woman seizing. On the monitor, she was found to be in ventricular fibrillation. Ventricular fibrillation is a lethal condition in which the heart's electrical conduction becomes disorganized and causes it to stop pumping blood. I immediately mobilized our team. CPR was started, and a shock was delivered with good improvement in the rhythm. I asked the triage nurse what the story was.

"This patient came in with chest pain . . . I think it's Dr. X's mom."

My heart sank. I took one look at her and knew she was critically ill. I began to treat her for a heart attack and cardiogenic shock, which can follow this condition. She was in respiratory distress and her breathing was labored. I knew she needed to be put on a ventilator. Dr. X ran in as I prepared to secure the patient's airway and prepare for intubation. She was expectedly distraught. She held her mom's hand and talked to her softly and tearfully.

I was lucky enough at this point to have a few wonderful colleagues now assisting me in the resuscitation. I successfully secured one of the most difficult airways in my life, and proceeded to place a large catheter into her neck so we could administer strong medications to help revive her heart. I called the cardiologist and begged them to take her for cardiac intervention. Eventually they did. I gave Dr. X a hug and wished her mom the best. She had been stabilized, but she was still critically ill.

As I returned to the emergency department, my mind wasn't right. But that didn't matter. I had many patients that needed my help and there was no one else to see them. I did the best I could to work through my distracted mind, but I was so focused on Dr. X and her mother that I could barely focus on the patients in front of me. Yet, patients continued to arrive and I continued to push. Sayings like "the show must go on" and "the curtain rises even on an actor's worst day," ran through my head. So I pushed through.

PERSPECTIVE

A few hours later, Dr. X came to me and said her mother was doing better. She required a cardiac stent and a machine called a "balloon pump," but she had stabilized, and many were optimistic. Dr. X gave me a big hug and I felt on top of the world. I thanked her for the good news, and she headed back to her mother's bedside. Meanwhile, I felt a new sense of energy and adrenaline. This is why I chose emergency medicine. I wanted to make a difference. I also loved that feeling of gratitude. Part of it felt selfish because that gratitude was euphoric.

As I was finishing my shift and getting ready to head home, Dr. X came back to my unit, more teary-eyed and visibly upset.

"It's over. She died. They tried their best, but she kept going in and out of ventricular fibrillation. They even let her wake up so I could say goodbye. We withdrew care and let her die peacefully."

Sadness pummeled me as I gave Dr. X a hug and my condolences. Logically, I knew she was critically ill, but still there was a part of me that felt like a failure. I let down my colleague and friend. As I walked back to my office to gather my belongings and head home, I kept it together, but once I got into my car, I rested my head on the steering wheel and my thoughts raced: *Did I not resuscitate her quickly enough? Could I have gotten to her side sooner? Did I give her the right medications? What could I have done differently?*

I had experienced a lot of death up to that point in my career. Rarely was I emotional or affected by the death of my patients, but Dr. X's mother was different. This was a colleague's mother. I would see her regularly and know she died after she was under my care. This was hard to deal with. The drive home was long and dispirited. I began to question my ability as a physician. When I got home, I emailed my two supportive colleagues who assisted in the management of Dr. X's mother and thanked them for being there for me. They wrote back extremely kind and encouraging words. Their words helped ease my mind slightly that evening.

The next day, the announcement was made to the department that Dr. X's mother had died, and funeral arrangements were provided. I had a few days off before the wake and I spent those days mostly trying to keep my mind off her mom. I spent the day exercising, walking at the park, going out to dinner. But I was uneasy. When my mind was idle, negative thoughts crept in. *How was the family? Did they blame me for not being able to ensure her survival? Did they want to see me at the wake?* All of these thoughts raced in my mind as I nervously purchased flowers to bring to the funeral home.

Once I arrived, I walked around and looked at the pictures of Dr. X and her family—all the memories they created over the years. To see all the smiling faces in the pictures, now teary-eyed and somber as they mourned the passing of their mother, was heartbreaking. I slowly crept into line to pay my respects and offer my condolences. When I eventually made it to Dr. X with apprehension, she reached out to me and gave me a firm hug.

"I'm sorry," I said softly.

"Thank you for giving me the chance to say goodbye to my mom. I will never forget that." Dr. X whispered in my ear.

She introduced me to her sister who also hugged and thanked me. I walked out of the funeral home and headed straight to my car. For some reason, I cried the whole way home despite the sudden feeling of a massive weight lifted off my shoulders. I needed those words to put me at ease and provide me peace. At that moment, I realized what it meant to be an emergency physician. Up until that point, my perspective had been completely wrong.

End-of-life care is as important as the beginning and the middle. It provides loved ones with peace. My efforts allowed Dr. X to give her mother a kiss and say goodbye prior to her death. And my efforts allowed her to die in a peaceful and controlled manner with her loved ones by her side. I have been extremely cognizant of how people die after caring for Dr. X's mother. To this day, I have never expressed gratitude to Dr. X for teaching me about humility, perspective, and the impact that even imperfect endings can have on people.

SIUH EAST: A COVID FIELD HOSPITAL ON STATEN ISLAND

DR. JEREL CHACKO AND DR. ERIC CIOE-PENA

WRITTEN FROM DR. CIOE-PENA'S PERSPECTIVE

The impact of the pandemic on healthcare systems world-wide has been immense, causing an unprecedented strain on medical facilities and personnel. Hospitals struggled to accommodate the surge of patients. Healthcare workers faced long hours, emotional turmoil, and an increased risk of contracting the virus themselves. In this grueling environment, the ability to adapt and innovate became critical, as healthcare professionals sought new ways to deliver care and protect both patients and staff from the virus.

As a global health doctor and emergency medicine physician, I vividly remember being bombarded nearly nonstop with calls from the emergency operation center in January of 2020 during my visit to our satellite facility in Ecuador. The confusion was palpable, given that the majority of our staff hadn't traveled in or around China, except for one doctor visiting family there. While health professionals in Ecuador were fretting about the possibility of coronavirus spreading to South America, I brushed off their anxiety as premature. Little did I know that in less than two months, I'd be thrown into the eye of the storm as the first wave of COVID-19 hit New York City.

I bounced around emergency departments, helping overwhelmed staff at Forest Hills Hospital cope with the chaos that unfolded. I've seen many crowded emergency departments in the United States, but none were as overrun as Forest Hills Hospital was in mid to late March 2020. The line of patients gasping for breath, waiting to be triaged by the nurse in the emergency department, spilled out into the ambulance bay. It was like nothing I'd ever seen before.

Each shift we saw more COVID than the last. It became clear that what started as an epidemic primarily focused in Queens was now spreading into Staten Island and Manhattan, according to news reports and colleagues' testimonials.

On Friday, April 3rd, 2020, I was working a shift at Staten Island University Hospital Prince's Bay when my phone rang. It was the Associate Chair of the emergency department, Dr. Joseph Basile, and my former boss, now the Executive Director of Staten Island University Hospital, Dr. Brahim Ardolic.

"We don't have enough space at the main campus— do you think we can make [the] South Beach [Psychiatric Facility] a field hospital?"

Dr. Ardolic had faith in my abilities, especially when it comes to working in limited-resource settings, so he asked me to help him set up the facility. This would require my undivided attention, expertise, and determination. Despite numerous challenges, I was committed to getting the job done right. The huge work at hand was exploring how emergency medicine could break the standard rules of medicine and achieve the primary goal of saving lives.

According to state regulations, the rooms in a hospital that treats COVID patients should be designed with enough ventilators, hospital beds, and healthcare personnel—but all those requisites were absent in the space. The physical infrastructure of a psychiatric facility is meant to maintain the safety of patients who are having mental health crises, not strains on their physical bodies. As such, the rooms are designed to reduce the risk of self-harm or harm against others, not for what is best to support the care of critically ill patients. This required prompt remodeling of the health organization's internal and external structure to ensure (1) proper ventilation and filtration, (2) awareness of clinical deterioration, (3) patient comfort and protection against harm, and (4) access to medical supplies.

Airborne Infection and Isolation Rooms (AIIR, or negative pressure rooms) are ideal for suspected or confirmed COVID patients, as the virus spreads more easily in an airtight environment. No infrastructure existed to support the adequate number of air exchanges per hour to contain viral spread. To optimize ventilation, we ensured that all recirculated air was filtered through viral filtration systems like HEPA and used mixed mechanical and natural ventilation schemes to achieve as close to twelve air changes per hour (ACH) as possible.

Another challenge was the need for awareness and responsiveness to patients' conditions, which was hindered by locked doors and the lack of an integrated call bell system. A call bell system in hospitals connects immobile or disabled patients to the nursing station and is crucial for urgent responses from medical personnel. It is a source of relief for vulnerable patients and can be the difference between life and death. The system helps alert caregivers to attend to patients and prevent worsening conditions. We deployed physical bells to act in lieu of an electronic alert system and took the doors off the hinges to ensure our nurses could purposefully round and reduce harmful events, such as falls or respiratory distress.

Hospital beds are essential for patients with emergency health conditions, as they are designed with special features such as CPR release, IV poles with hooks, detachable head and footboards, and built-in nursing controls to provide better and constant care to the patient. Guidelines by the Department of Health and Social Care emphasize the need for electricity operation, adjustable positioning, and pressure relief mattresses. These features all work to reduce the risk of injury and allow for patients' bodily functions. Unfortunately, these beds would not fit in the field hospital rooms, so we utilized the next best option—hospital stretchers.

SIUH EAST: A COVID FIELD HOSPITAL ON STATEN ISLAND

Hospitals need to always have key medical equipment on hand to provide comprehensive care. In addition to stretchers, this list includes defibrillators, anesthesia machines, patient monitors, sterilizers, EKG/ECG machines, surgical tables, blanket and fluid warmers, electrosurgical units, and surgical lights. In addition to the standard medical apparatuses, certain equipment is necessary for an acute COVID room, such as gloves, medical face masks, ventilators, oxygen humidifiers, flow-splitters, laryngoscopes, infusion pumps, and COVID-19 test kits. Other necessary devices for acute COVID hospitals include hemofiltration equipment and sets, active humidifiers, suction devices, CRP and other markers of inflammation tests, blood gas analyzers, tubes for nasopharyngeal swabs, viral transport medium, and nucleic acid extraction kits. Much of which we were severely lacking.

To tackle this deficiency, we implemented various strategies, including transferring equipment and supplies from non-essential departments to our COVID field hospital, making agreements with authorities and suppliers to access institutional and central reserves, and prioritizing network management for procurement. We established a physical space within the hospital for storing additional supplies while factoring in easy access, safety, temperature, ventilation, exposure to light, and moisture levels. Moreover, we had to carefully manage the allocation of resources, ensuring that we had adequate supplies of personal protective equipment (PPE) to keep our staff safe. This required us to establish a

PPE conservation program, closely monitor usage, and make adjustments to our protocols to minimize waste.

The ability to adapt and innovate was crucial in this context, as we sought to balance the need for effective infection control measures with the limited availability of essential resources. We tackled the lack of wall oxygen and suction by leveraging oxygen concentrators to extract oxygen from the air and control its delivery for the treatment of hypoxemia in COVID patients and deploying portable suction machines.

Even with the building being remodeled and retrofitted to support acute-care services, we still had challenges with staffing on all ends—physicians, physician extenders, and nurses. We were able to leverage our membership within a larger health system, Northwell Health, by using the Northwell in-house agency nursing to help support staffing while also utilizing nurses from redeployed departments and locations. On top of the ongoing redeployment of physician extender staff (i.e. physician assistants and nurse practitioners), extra part-time or temporary staff were recruited to meet the rising demands. We set up a training program to educate these new staff members on COVID-19 care protocols and the specific challenges of working in a field hospital setting. This allowed us to establish a cohesive team that was well prepared to handle the unique circumstances we faced.

On top of the basic patient care environments being set up to support the clinical teams, patients admitted for COVID-19 presented a unique challenge in that, while these patients were in general hemodynamically stable and not requiring intensive care unit (ICU) monitoring, a single physiological variable—the patient's blood oxygen saturation (SpO2) level—was something that could be labile and required monitoring at a frequency above what typical Med-Surg units could deliver. Dr. Jerel Chacko was instrumental in assuring that instead of overutilizing ICU spaces to deliver the higher frequency of SpO2 checks, we deployed a novel wearable technology, the BioBeat wearable chest monitor. This was a small module that adhered to a patient's chest, allowing for continuous and remote viewing of the patient's heart rate, blood oxygen saturation, respiratory rate, blood pressure, and temperature. This allowed for a reduction in PPE waste and contagion exposure, as these vital signs could be collected in real-time on-demand without the need to physically go into the room. The closer eye on the monitor paired with both automated alerting and manual alerting by a partnership with a remote TeleHealth team, located out in Long Island, allowed a higher level of safety than typically found in a Med-Surg unit.

TeleHealth infrastructure was also advantageous to COVID patients, as we were able to deploy two video-enabled carts to our field hospital, which enabled patients to obtain consultation by physicians who did not need to travel to provide in-person care and did not need to expose themselves to contagion. Without these carts, patients would potentially need to be moved to obtain specialty consultation. This technology reduced the burden on a stressed EMS system.

In addition to these innovative solutions, we recognized the importance of supporting the mental well-being of our healthcare workers who were on the frontlines, battling the pandemic day in and day out. The emotional toll of the crisis was significant, and it was essential to address the mental health needs of our staff. We provided access to counseling services, stress management workshops, and peer support programs. We also coordinated with other hospitals, non-profit organizations, and government bodies to share information and resources. Partnerships like these played a crucial role in the rapid response to the pandemic. These actions were important in helping our team maintain their resilience and continue providing the best possible care to our patients.

The field hospital was operational for several months, providing care to hundreds of patients during the peak of the pandemic in New York City. It also eased the pressure on the main hospitals, allowing them to focus on non-COVID cases and continue providing essential services to the community. We learned valuable lessons about adapting quickly, working under extreme pressure, and managing resources in times of crisis.

As the COVID-19 pandemic continues to evolve and new variants emerge, the experiences from setting up and running the field hospital at South Beach Psychiatric Facility can serve as a model for future emergency response efforts. The ability to rapidly transform spaces into medical facilities and organize staffing, supplies, and equipment will remain an essential skill in healthcare.

Our efforts in creating the field hospital were a testament to the power of innovation and determination in the face of adversity. We drew upon our collective knowledge and experience, as well as the spirit of collaboration and resourcefulness that is at the heart of emergency medicine, to overcome the many challenges that arose during the transformation of the psychiatric facility and thus saved countless lives. By pooling our resources and expertise, we were able to provide care for those in need during one of the most challenging times in modern history.

As we move forward, the lessons learned from this experience will undoubtedly shape our approach to future healthcare crises and reinforce the importance of preparedness, adaptability, and resilience. The experience of setting up and running the field hospital at South Beach Psychiatric Facility also underscores the importance of ongoing investment in public health infrastructure and emergency preparedness. The COVID-19 pandemic has highlighted the vulnerabilities in our healthcare systems and demonstrated the need for robust, adaptable, and well-resourced public health strategies. By learning from our experiences during this crisis, we can better prepare for future emergencies and work toward building more resilient and responsive healthcare systems that can withstand the challenges of the twenty-first century.

A TEAM SPORT WITH GREAT TEAMWORK

Dr. Paul Barbara

The game of baseball was a constant in my house growing up. The innumerable pop culture references to the connections that baseball—or many other organized sports—provides in a family are proof of how vital these activities are to human resiliency. One line in the movie *City Slickers* references how Daniel Stern's character could "always talk with [his] Dad about baseball, no matter what else might have been going on." This quote rang true in my house, baseball was always a regularity that we could talk about even if an argument was ongoing.

As a young man I wanted to play centerfield for my hometown New York Yankees. I soon came to realize that occupational training was more relevant to my future growth and any family members of mine. I was fifteen years old when I told my parents I wanted to enter medicine. The year was

1992, and I had no idea what my future life would hold, but I was raised in a house built on optimism and initiative. The tenets of my career choice were based around job security, community service, and a personal commitment to science. Centerfield might've been out of reach, but ironically my future baseball experiences would eventually affirm this career choice in medicine.

While attending college, I went to EMT school, finally procuring my blue cargo work pants and a pair of black work boots, thus beginning a long career in emergency medicine. We trained, went on calls, provided care, learned from local paramedics how to interact with patients and local hospitals, washed the vehicles. A common theme in this country is the difficulty its providers find in crafting a long career. For me, EMS was always a steppingstone to medical school and beyond. I always endeavored to honor those who didn't have the same opportunities by furthering my career beyond the back of the rig.

My residency training in Emergency Medicine was completed soon thereafter at The Brooklyn Hospital Center. Naturally, post-graduation I sought out additional training in Emergency Medical Services, and secured post graduate education in EMS, a newly recognized specialty of emergency medicine. By 2015, I had become well established as an attending physician in my hometown at Staten Island University Hospital.

However, my greatest save in the ER wasn't in a hospital at all. Ironically, it started with me in the centerfield region of a Little League baseball diamond.

A TEAM SPORT WITH GREAT TEAMWORK

My wife and I wanted to instill the same love of baseball in our household, so I volunteered to coach our son's Little League team. As always, I kept quiet about my occupation, as it had no bearing on my role as a coach. I found that baseball's ability to bring people together, at least until the game starts, had endured through my years away studying medicine. When I took the coaching job, I also wanted to continue to strengthen the bonds growing between our six-year-old son and me, but never did I anticipate that I would need to employ my emergency medicine expertise in front of him and his teammates.

On April 18, 2015, I was simply an under-slept "Dad Coach." Opening Day of the local Little League began with a parade through the town and was followed by ceremonies and invocations for the entire league. Our team was staged in the centerfield area, many of the players and parents meeting for the first time. Shortly after the national anthem concluded and during a local politician's invocation, a commotion ensued in the third-base dugout. The shadows were playing typical tricks, but from where I was, I thought I saw a man collapse. My blue Under Armour athletic shirt would have to suffice for scrubs. I hopped past another coach and sped to the dugout. Retrospectively, I question the instinctual sprint, but it's now evident to me that these are the situations where we find out that the career chooses the provider. My role was about to make itself incredibly evident.

A fifty-two-year-old man was in cardiac arrest. Unbeknownst to me, he was a leader at the Local Little

League, a long-tenured coach and board member who had coached countless children and was even part of the Little League World Series team from Staten Island years prior. I had no knowledge of his standing nor how he was felt to be family by so many of the Little League members. I just found him gasping and choking on the ground. I quickly introduced myself to the bystanders and one of his colleagues mentioned "cardiac patient" with an expected level of panic.

My first instinct was that he went into a rapid decompensation of heart failure, which can sometimes be alleviated by repositioning the patient, so I tried to prop him up. My instincts were in fact incorrect, but I was fortunate to have an unexpected teammate clarify how erroneous my initial judgment was.

As I continued in my futility of repositioning the patient—whom I thought was still alive—to augment breathing, an off-duty FDNY Captain/Baseball Dad presented himself to the clamor. We had never met, but he spoke clearly above the cacophony and said plainly: "Doc . . . he's gone."

While his statement was temporarily true, many of us knew the next steps to take. I am thankful this person provided clarity to redirect my adrenaline-infused bias and help me see the event as an evolving life-and-death situation. I arrived at the scene so promptly that I was blinded to the fact that the patient was actually in cardiac arrest.

Cardiac arrest scientists have now categorized what I witnessed, agonal gasps, as one of the first signs of a patient going into cardiac arrest. Agonal gasps are now a threshold for everyone, laypersons as well as medical professionals, to initiate the healthcare response cascade including 911 activation and delivery of rescue devices like automated external defibrillators.

Continuing this cognitive pivot and considering the resources available in the moment, I stepped back from his side.

"OK, let's work him. Right here."

Just like any hackneyed public safety video, I began chest compressions, gloveless, then made deliberate eye contact with an unknown at the dugout fence, and started calling out directions:

"YOU. CALL 911."

"YOU. GET AN AED."

There was no standby unit, first aid squad, or organized event medical response at this large gathering. I continued calling out orders to nameless faces of the volunteer responders—all coaches, parents, or members of the Little League. Our multiagency, multidisciplinary, multigenerational, actually, just plain motley crew of rescuers likely had facial recognition of their teammates, but to date none had ever worked a cardiac arrest patient together. We went about our business, seamlessly efficient despite an absence of prior collaboration. When friends ask me "how I get through [blank]," my answer is always the same: "together." However, teams aren't always who you show up at work with. Hidden teams are out there, with all the right people, waiting for an emergent situation of need to present itself.

Eventually, as more people came to help, I found myself standing on the dugout bench to maximize my vantage, facilitate our goals, and enhance provider safety during care as the resuscitation continued. Only later did we find out the responders were off-duty police officers, firefighters, nurses, physician assistants, or even medical laypeople who just wanted to help the cause. This event demonstrated an epitome of Staten Island that I've always believed in: We're a group of people who can serve their neighbors 24/7.

We continued compressions, alternating providers. My coaching partner reluctantly came to the dugout for a status update, with my only request being to hold on to my son in the interim, thus becoming "Uncle Dom" to this day. An AED arrived from an off-duty NYPD squad car. In the hands of a capable municipal response member, prompt rhythm assessment demonstrated the benefits of our chest compressions, that the patient was actually in a shockable rhythm, something that we could act upon right here from the dugout. Not all patients in cardiac arrest have the type of rhythm that an AED can defibrillate. These real-life situations contrast the pop culture analogies of the patient being miraculously saved by this cardiac defibrillation, commonly known as a shock. Some of the cardiac arrest patients that EMS encounters are not found quickly enough for the AED to be able to shock the patient back into a normal rhythm.

SHOCK ADVISED

He couldn't press the orange button fast enough, but thankfully a boisterous call to clear the patient was made, averting any additional crises such as an accidental provider shock from the chaos. The first defibrillation provided a return of spontaneous circulation to the patient. His heart was beating and his body was beginning to restore its normal functions. We had a pulse, but our patient remained comatose. He needed critical care management and likely an emergency cardiac intervention.

The closest hospital was a community facility, and not equipped with emergent cardiac intervention capability. Naturally, the local EMS protocol was to take this patient to the closest hospital. However, EMS protocols can't possibly be written to account for every life (and death) situation. My final cognitive pivot would be to take a chance for this man and his family and get him to the facility with interventional cardiac capability. The only problem was, I had no rights to do that. People like me have no official field response capability for my hospital or the NYC 911 system.

However, as I had trained in this very system several years prior, I knew the way to make it work. While he was being prepared by the now on-scene EMS crews, I made calls to the NYC Medical Control physician and requested for the approval for the crew to take him to the longer-distanced, yet potentially lifesaving, tertiary care facility. Little did I know the off-duty and now on-duty police cars present had silently organized to provide a full escort for the ambulance bearing our patient. Time and distance would become relatively malleable with green lights the whole way, and he made it successfully to the ED and onto the cardiac catheterization lab, where the lifesaving work continued by the next member of the team.

Our patient lived through this ordeal, and we were able to be reunited with him after his recuperation. Fortunately, the lifesaving event and its influence had not yet concluded. A local sports-radio broadcaster was silently in the audience that day as part of these opening events that were interrupted by the medical emergency. The story was discussed that Monday morning during drive-time on the local sports media channel, WFAN, by radio jockeys Boomer Esiason and Craig Carton.

Other news media and the hospital public relations ran this feel-good story for the typical seventy-two-hour news cycle, often reaching out for a quote or a soundbite. We were able to utilize this platform to push awareness for public access defibrillation, field medical response, and the importance of situational awareness for all in youth sports. Although "the doctor" was often the focus in these media stories, I assure all readers that the real saviors on the field were the immediate collective of like-minded individuals focusing on a common mission: helping this person. Those who answered the call that day demonstrated their duty to love an unknowing victim.

This interaction reaffirmed so many concepts about Emergency Medicine and its importance in our individual communities. It also allowed me to negotiate equipping my car with an AED. Happily, my employer obliged, and it remains unused to date other than school demonstrations for classes our son or daughters attend.

Fortunately, there aren't any more cardiac arrest stories for this Dad / Hockey Coach / Physician. In reflection, I'm thankful that my career allows me to give back to my family and others. Chaotic events like this can provide a sense of purpose and clarity to emergency healthcare providers such as myself and the others that participated in this out-of-hospital cardiac arrest resuscitation. There is an emotional and cognitive reward to know that our training and professional diligence can have an impact beyond the traditional occupational arena. Most importantly, this experience validated that being part of a team does not always mean wearing a jersey or keeping score.

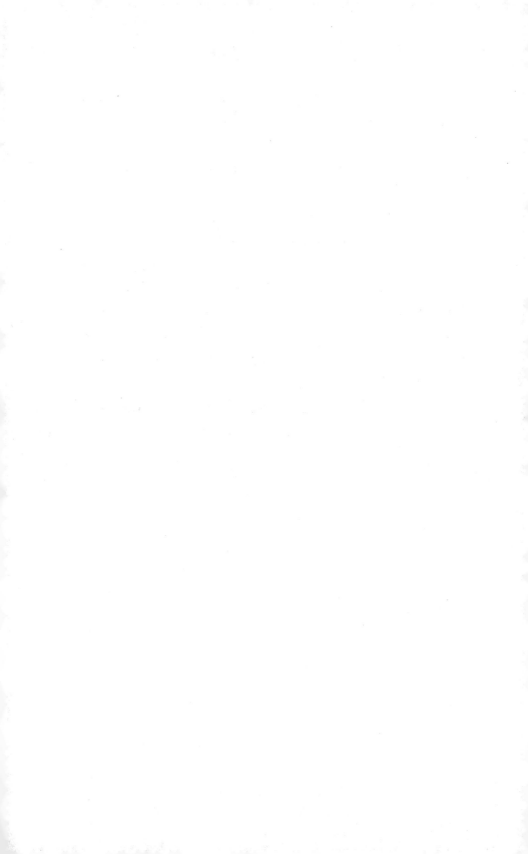

TELLING SOMEONE THEY'RE DYING

Dr. Brahim Ardolic

"I'm sure you don't remember me."

"I remember you. I told your mother she had cancer."

I remembered her because giving bad news is something I have had to do often in my career, and I can say I remember most of them vividly.

Whenever people ask about healthcare as a career option for themselves or, most commonly, their children, I will often respond with this question: Why are you, or your family member, considering a career in healthcare? This will usually lead to a list of reasons that rarely include caring for people. If they make it to a third reason and haven't talked about the patient, this profession might not be the right fit.

In order to *take care* of people, you need to *care* about people. It is easy to care about doing a good job, or even care about coming to the rescue. Medical school is full of overachievers that want to succeed at all costs. There are many good doctors who are efficient and take great care of their patients. There are fewer great doctors who really care about the human beings they are taking care of.

I have managed large groups of healthcare providers for many years and watched many careers begin. You know how a provider will perform once you see them interact with people. Residency is excellent at producing technically skilled, affable people who are excellent at their jobs. For many doctors, it is also effective at dehumanizing patients. Every physician feels the first time they experience a death, but imagine knowing that even if you did your job perfectly, a certain number of people were going to die, either in front of you or very soon after they leave your care. Imagine being a mechanic and knowing that even if every car you fix is perfect, one in one hundred will blow up in a few hours. Would you be so quick to get to know the drivers?

Healthcare providers are often divided into two groups: those who distance themselves from their patients, and those who lean into their patients and care even more. If you meet the latter, consider them a keeper.

They teach you a lot of things in medical school and residency:

They teach you how to recognize disease.

They teach you how to treat disease.

They even teach you a fair amount about human interactions.

Unfortunately, as a doctor, your education is often learned

on the fly, and is designed to teach you efficiency, not human-ism. Specifically, there is little or no training on giving good and bad news, and no training on dealing with how caught up you really get in people's lives in that one brief encounter. You see a lot of people at one of the worst moments in their life. You tell them they just had a massive heart attack, or that they have a ruptured intestine or an aneurysm in their brain and need to go to the OR immediately to have it repaired, or that you have no idea what's wrong with them, even though they're extremely frightened and want answers.

There are some interactions, however, that are on a com-pletely different level. Only two types of news are worse than just about anything else you could tell a person, and sadly, most doctors have to deliver both many times.

First is telling someone their loved one has died. And sec-ond is telling a patient they have a terminal illness. Nothing compares. These two situations are so hard because of how we grieve as humans. When you walk into a room and tell someone that their loved one is gone or that they are never going to recover from this disease you just diagnosed, you are often taking them from a regular day in their life to an unimaginable situation.

When you ask someone what the hardest part of dealing with a terminal illness is, they always say "getting used to the idea" and their family's acceptance. Here, in one horrible moment, as the doctor, you have to confront both: You have to tell someone to get used to the idea that they are dying, and it's usually in the presence of a loved one.

One of the things that's wrong with healthcare is that most people are bad at having that conversation, or they are simply unwilling to. Therefore, so many people wind up with false expectations. For example: Many of you have had a loved one with cancer. How many of you had a loved one who needed a second course of treatment because the cancer recurred? Do you know that, with certain very specific exceptions, a recurrence of cancer after an initial treatment will wind up being terminal? Did you know that, barring certain exceptions, care becomes about extending life and not about curing? I'm not saying this is a bad thing, because we can do some truly amazing things now to extend people's lives, but do those patients and families know that a cure is essentially out of the equation? In my experience, they don't. Now don't get me wrong, I'm not a fatalist in any way. I am, however, a strong believer in helping people understand what's exactly happening.

Yes, I remember this daughter very well. When you take care of people for a living, you meet many concerned relatives. This daughter was memorable for many reasons. First, she looked very much like a younger version of her mom. She was concerned that her mother was minimizing her symptoms. I could tell she was very worried, and that this was more serious than the mother thought. So, these two friendly faces—a mirror with two decades in between—were easy to remember.

It was around 10:00 o'clock in the morning, and I was the attending on call in the medical emergency department.

I was working with a wonderful senior resident. The resident presented a case to me that I had heard many times in the past, but this one sounded slightly more concerning than most. She presented a woman in her early sixties who had been having a cough for quite some time. The patient had been a smoker for many years, but quit a few months ago. She said that she had seen her doctor three times for the cough and was just feeling tired.

She noted that the patient had completed two courses of antibiotics for what had been described as an upper respiratory infection. Her previous exams were unremarkable each time, her blood counts were in normal range, and her chest x-ray was read as negative. Her doctor had also referred her to a pulmonologist, with whom she had an appointment in four weeks.

The patient's daughter was concerned by her mother's lack of appetite and weight loss and didn't want to wait a month to find out if her mom had emphysema, so they came to the ER. After talking to the resident and asking specific questions about the exam, I entered Room 5 and recall seeing a woman who looked as if she had recently lost a significant amount of weight.

I asked the patient and her daughter to tell us the whole story again. We do this to patients not to annoy them, but to help the resident learn, and because you can gather a lot more information this way. The patient confirmed my suspicion that she had not been trying to lose weight. At the end of each patient's description, I always ask the question: What are you most concerned about?

She told me she was worried she quit smoking too late, and she had lung cancer. By the time we got to that question, I was fairly certain she was right.

Too much evidence suggested she was ill. She clearly looked like somebody that was not thriving at home. She clearly looked older than her actual age. You can learn a lot from someone's skin color, too. Did you ever wonder why they often describe the healthy baby as having rosy cheeks? Or why skin care companies talk about a "healthy pink hue"? Sallow, mottled, pale, or pale-yellow skin is often a sign something is wrong. Especially if it is a real change from that person's usual coloration. Think about the last time you thought someone you know looked sick. What are you really seeing? Usually, you're responding to their facial expressions and skin coloration.

While my exam didn't really conclude much other than mild wheezing consistent with early emphysema, I was worried enough that I wanted to see her chest CT before she went home. Usually, I would recommend the scan be performed in an outpatient facility, but I didn't know her doctor and she didn't have a follow-up visit scheduled for a month. I had no illusions about what I was going to find in the cat scan of the chest. I was convinced I would get a normal blood panel, a normal chest x-ray, and a really bad CT.

There are many times as a doctor that you really want to be wrong. It's your job to worry about people, and you love nothing more than being worried and then being wrong. I really wish I had been wrong here. Her blood was fine; her chest x-ray was not normal, but not terrible. Her chest CT showed a very large tumor in the middle of her chest that wasn't showing up on x-ray because of her heart. A huge blow. Not just because it was clearly cancer, but because it was likely advanced stage 4 cancer. The tumor was likely Small Cell Carcinoma and would take her life. I had to decide how to react.

A lot of doctors, based upon their own discomfort, end up giving vague answers to patients about what they see. In residency, I had seen one of my attendings tell a mom that her teenager had been killed. His delivery of the news was so confusing that I wasn't sure the child had died.

From that point on, I promised myself that I would never shirk the responsibility of giving my patients or their families bad news. I owed it to them to take their cases seriously and to own the moment. Not because I felt I was so good at it; but because I watched so many people be so bad at providing accurate information to patients while acknowledging the sensitivity of the situation and the associated pain. I would take full responsibility and never leave these families not fully understanding what they had been told.

Until you've actually witnessed a parent having the realization that they have lost their child, you don't truly understand what the toll of gun violence is. Sadly, because I trained during the tail end of the crack epidemic in Brooklyn, I have seen those numerous times. I was a party to that conversation or had that conversation more times than I can count. I remember more about every time I had to tell a parent or a loved one that they lost a young person than all the good cases I treated. All the saves, the diagnostic dilemmas, the unusual cases that make you think—they all are forgotten compared to the anguish of a family who loses someone too young. The faces of every single mom and dad, whose hearts I broke, are imprinted in my brain, even after all these years.

The look of unexpected terrible sadness is actually very hard to describe. Once you have seen it, you know what it looks like and never forget. The forlorn parent has a look of anguish that is carried by everyone that sees it. I sadly see it in the media after mass shootings, especially those involving minors. They are hard for me to look at because of how often I have seen those faces in person.

That's what was on my mind after the CT scan, when I prepared to deliver the news to this woman and to her daughter.

I made a point of bringing the resident with me. The more the doctor in training is exposed to doctors who understand how difficult and important this is, the better. Like all learning points, you hope to pass this forward to the next generation of doctors. If you can help one trainee, you are helping the one hundred thousand patients she or he will treat over a thirty-year career. That's right, the average ED doc will treat around one hundred thousand patients in their career. Think about all the people who you will never meet but can be helped by this one person you taught!

We spent about fifteen minutes with the patient's daughter talking about what we had found. If you understand emergency medicine, you understand how precious those fifteen minutes are and how many things need to happen, but there are things you just can't rush. Certain things that just take time. We talked about the fact that we had found a mass in her lungs and that it was in a concerning location. I informed her that, while I couldn't definitely tell her that she had cancer, this would require further workup and would likely be cancer.

She passed away four months after we had met—when I told her she likely had small cell cancer of the lung.

You really only get to give a couple of kinds of good news in emergency medicine, and they are usually wrapped around bad news.

"Yes, your significant other is still alive. We were able to get them to the operating room or Cath lab or whatever in time."

"Yes, we were able to get your significant other's heart restarted after giving them X, Y, and Z and now they're going to the ICU, so we can only hope for the best."

It's the kind of news that is always tinged with concern, and sometimes around regret. At the end of the day, it's very easy as an ER doctor to treat the person's body and never truly recognize the impact that you can make on someone's life by taking the time and having the kindness to be able to do something the right way.

So, you can imagine, when a random waitress walks up to you while you are having breakfast at a diner and asks if you remember her, it isn't usually a good thing. This is especially true when a family member comes up to you and asks you about a case that occurred in the distant past. When I remembered telling her mother that she was likely terminally ill, I can't say I wasn't worried that somehow I had done something wrong or there was a complication I had overlooked.

Usually, the next sentence isn't a happy one, but what she said to me is something that I will carry for the rest of my life.

"I just wanted to thank you. We knew that this was cancer the moment you started talking. You took it so seriously. She went to other physicians that beat around the bush and told her that there were ways to treat her knowing full well this was really aggressive and the options were incredibly limited. Thanks for preparing us."

I never got to tell her how much it meant to me that she thanked me or how much it shaped future interactions. I went and found the resident to make sure that the resident knew that I had been thanked and that she had been thanked, and that she should also remember the case.

Who would ever have thought that my most memorable case is a woman who I couldn't save?

I never believed that you have to become hardened as a physician to deal with all of the sadness you see. I always tried to show kindness and compassion to every person, especially those who had terminal illnesses. Knowing this daughter saw that, and understood I was trying to help even when I couldn't, still means the world to me. That confirmation helped me more than I was ever able to help her mom.

UNITY IN THE FACE OF CHAOS

DR. SHOROK HASSAN AND DR. DANIELLE LANGAN

Working in the emergency room is a day-to-day mystery and we are taught to expect the unexpected. We thrive in an environment surrounded by a team of individuals who cultivate trust and support so we can handle whatever walks through our door. Although each team member offers a different perspective on patient care, the way everyone can prioritize their responsibilities and come together is what makes working in the emergency room so special.

Although the chaos and excitement are what draws people in to work in this field, it can be overwhelming to see the broad spectrum of patient presentations. You are exposed to various medical specialties in the emergency room, and each patient's case becomes more intense than the next.

Many emergency providers can relate to working a busy shift and can often easily recall that one shift that will stick with them forever, no matter how many new cases arise. We will never forget a shift we had together; the severity and volume of patients seemed to stand out that day: a toxicologic overdose case in one room, a cardiac arrest occurring next door, a stroke code across the hall, a cardiac patient requiring BiPAP, multiple patients from a high-speed motor vehicle collision, a gunshot wound, and an airway-compromising throat infection with airway setup on standby. But amongst all this, one patient will remain imprinted in our minds.

The following case remains a mystery to this day. We do not know what caused the following events to occur, and we likely never will. Being in different phases of your career, cases like this help you realize the importance of good training and how the relationships and trust formed amongst the team make all the difference when a critical patient arrives unexpectedly. Let's look at the case through the eyes of the resident versus attending physician.

* * *

The Resident: Picture the attending physician rolling in a patient slumped over in a wheelchair who was unresponsive. Seeing this, I had no idea what to expect. I followed them into an open resuscitation room. Without hesitation, an all-female team of the attending, two of our nurses, and I lifted this patient together onto a clean stretcher. We knew this resuscitation was going to be an all-hands-on-deck situation. As the attending communicated the next steps, the unthinkable happened: the patient's entire face and body became entirely swollen and went from pale to blue to purple prior to an attempt at intubation. This meant I had to perform my first surgical airway. My fears slowly subsided as I looked at my attending who was commanding the room with confidence and poise. Additionally, one of our oral-maxillofacial surgeons was right beside me, prepared to assist at every juncture.

With all this support, I knew I was ready. And although the procedure was conducted successfully, we were unable to keep our patient alive after an arduous resuscitation. This tragedy felt as if it occurred in the blink of an eye. After their death, our patient's spouse arrived at the emergency department. When we broke the news, the spouse said they were not surprised by the events. The spouse knew their partner was not taking care of their health for a long time, having not seen a healthcare provider for many years. Still, they expressed nothing but gratitude for our team's resuscitation efforts. As a healthcare provider, we know that nothing will ever make this conversation less heartbreaking.

* * *

The Attending: As the attending physician, it is important to remain astute and meticulous, while still overseeing everything that is happening on the shift. As I rolled that patient in that wheelchair, slumped over, and initially pale, I knew I had to keep my composure for the sake of the patient and team. Panic only creates chaos. It is important to maintain confidence and calmness every step of the way.

The minute my team saw me wheeling the patient into

the room, they immediately rushed over and assisted me in lifting the patient onto the bed. Within seconds, a seamless step-by-step approach with excellent communication of events took place. As this patient was in cardiac arrest, I was leading the resuscitation, standing at the base of the bed. My role in those never-forgotten minutes was to lead my team, assigning specific tasks and ensuring completion. The role I knew would be most challenging was that of the airway. The patient quickly became edematous. The look of fear over-came the faces of my team, especially the senior resident who was preparing to secure the airway in the next few seconds. I looked back at her and reminded her she could handle this.

As the supervising physician, people look to you for that confidence and reassurance. Providing her with those words would help ease her fears and get her into a confident mind-set to successfully secure this airway. Also completing my emergency medicine residency at SIUH, I was familiar with the training this resident had received and was confident she would be successful. I was once that resident standing at the head of the bed about to handle a difficult airway; now it was her turn. A cricothyroidotomy would be our next step.

Guiding my resident through these steps and reassuring her was key to the success of this airway. Of course, it was challenging while maintaining a slew of emotions of your own: your heart racing inside your chest, sweat rolling down your back; yet still maintaining the calm, addressing each member of the team, and reminding yourself how things will come together. Preparation, believing in yourself, believing in your team, and good training all ensure success. And so those negative feelings quickly become silenced, and your mind tackles the situation clearly and focused.

The resident locked eyes with me, grabbed the scalpel, and with the additional support of our oral maxillofacial team, she performed the procedure with excellence and precision: we had obtained return-of-spontaneous circulation within seconds. Although I knew this may not be sustained, as the patient had other complications, we walked away knowing we provided the best care possible.

* * *

Our job was not complete, however. The other component of being part of this team is the sorrowful conversation with the family. As I stood there with the husband of this patient, he looked at me and said we had provided the only care and support to his wife, as she had been ill for quite some time and sought no medical attention until this shift. He witnessed firsthand the incredible efforts of the team, praising our sincere desire to help, our communication, and our organizational skills. This spoke volumes. As fast as all this happened, looking back, seeing all the pieces in slow motion, you realize how each component plays a huge part in providing a bigger picture. Although a mystery, this case proved the importance of teamwork, communication, interdisciplinary support, compassion, and hard work.

Yes, this was a chaotic day, as some may put it, and chaos is often the only thing that is not a mystery in the emergency room. Sometimes we do not solve every case that presents itself to us, but the lesson learned from a case such as this one is the importance of acceptance and growth and sometimes that is the win. Although in the emergency department there are various roles, perspectives, and responsibilities, at the end of the day we always can rely on our heath care team to come together to provide unity in the face of chaos for our patients. When you know that you and your team worked together and did the right thing for the patient, it eases the burden of a difficult encounter.

Looking back on that day, we can both say that we are proud to be a part of the SIUH emergency department family. We were part of an all-female team of healthcare providers, working together during a particularly hectic shift to save a life. Furthermore, we were part of an interdisciplinary team. For example, our oral-maxillofacial surgeon rushed to the emergency department to assist with a life-saving airway intervention without hesitation. Even though not every case will be solved in our line of work, having unwavering support from a strong interdisciplinary team at SIUH can ease the feelings of uncertainty knowing optimal patient care is being provided. Uniting in our debriefing process after these challenging cases provides insight to how to better handle future mystery cases.

Medicine is not stagnant; it is an ever-growing process, constantly evolving. This transformative and often-challenging landscape shapes us into assiduous emergency medicine providers, proud of the work that we do and will continue to do for years to come.

THE TRAGIC, COMICAL, AND SOMETIMES RIDICULOUS ENCOUNTERS IN THE ER

Dr. Francis Sabatino

Over the years, certain stories stick out in my head. Some are incredibly tragic; others are comical and many can be ridiculous.

One of the most tragic occurred at the beginning of my career at a hospital in the Midwest—one of my first encounters with an ER patient. It was an average weekday in early fall; a Tuesday, if I remember correctly. The call came over the radio from an ambulance that was five minutes away from the hospital: a young patient in his early twenties, unresponsive and in cardiac arrest. Unfortunately, not entirely uncommon. As we prepared the critical care unit with the equipment we would need and mobilized staff, the patient arrived.

He was rolled into the emergency room on a stretcher. Everyone seemed to freeze as the reality of the situation crept from our eyes to our brains. The patient was knocked into the bottom of a corn silo by a piece of farming machinery and had to be pulled out after an unknown but considerable amount of time. CPR was in progress. We mobilized as quickly as we could.

The first step in virtually all resuscitation cases is to secure the airway. In this case, we would need to intubate the patient, which involves placing a breathing tube in his throat and using machines to help him breathe. What was unforgettable about him was that his nose and mouth were so densely packed with corn kernels that we had to shovel it out with our gloved hands by the handful. Corn was everywhere. It took an extended amount of time, but eventually we were able to pass a tube to breath for him. CPR continued and we administered medications to try to restart his heart. The chances of survival were essentially non-existent, but we kept trying.

Later, some of his family arrived. I saw the shock come over his father's eyes as he walked into the emergency room and saw his dead son covered in a mixture of blood, mud, dirt, corn, and other debris scattered throughout the room. It was truly heartbreaking and unbelievable.

While it has been more than a decade since this incident occurred, it still feels like it was yesterday. The insanity of the sight and smell of that room is etched into my permanent memory. I try to use this as a constant reminder that life as you know it can be permanently altered in mere seconds.

On any shift working in the emergency department, you have to be prepared to walk out of a room filled with the guttural wails of grieving family members over the sudden loss of a son or daughter and into a different room filled with a completely different situation.

During an ordinary, uneventful Sunday night shift in late summer, I was working with one of the best physician's assistants we have on staff. The tracking board showed two new patients with the same last name and the same complaint: Assault.

We walked into the room and found a mother and her son. The mother was around eighty years old and was the embodiment of an Italian grandmother. She spoke half English and half Italian, but only talked with her hands. She had curlers in her hair, and was wearing a sleeveless, red-flowered sundress that looked more like a robe. She had stockings on and wore old sandals. Her son was around sixty years old—average height and weight. He was wearing shorts, sandals, a t-shirt with cutoff sleeves, and held an ice pack to his forehead.

We started by trying to obtain a history and attempt to figure out what had happened. The son began by saying that his mother hit him in the head with a baseball bat and then things suddenly got interesting. Earlier in the night, she heard strange noises coming from the basement of her house. She went to inspect the noise and saw a bat flying around the hallway. To defend herself, she picked up a baseball bat and started swinging it to try to kill the bat. She was standing several steps from the top of a basement staircase, violently swinging a baseball bat trying to crush a bat. Nothing but swings and misses.

She must have let out a few loud screams because her son came to inspect the noise. As he opened the door to see what the cause of the commotion was, she swung the baseball bat. Instead of hitting the bat, she connected with her son's head. Dazed, her son collapsed from a head injury and rolled down the remainder of the steps.

The mother over-rotated on her swing and started to panic after her son fell down the steps, so then she lost her balance and also tumbled down the steps, landing on top of him. They both ended up at the base of the steps with head injuries.

At this point in the story, both the physician assistant and I could hardly keep ourselves from laughing. I recalled a similar scene from the 1988 movie *The Great Outdoors* with Dan Aykroyd and John Candy. In my head, I am hysterically laughing and picturing the mom and her son all geared up with a catcher's mask and tennis rackets trying to kill this bat!

Their treatment was pretty routine. We fixed the laceration on the son's head and performed head-injury protocols on the mother. Then, we obtained basic imaging with no suspicion of long-term or complicating injuries on either patient. I expected an uneventful discharge, then the unthinkable happened. As we walked back in the room to update the patient, she opens her bag and states, "Oh, I also have the bat, if you want to see it."

I turned in disbelief and did a few double takes. It honestly took me a few minutes to process the information. Sure enough, she opens her bag and there is a bat in a zip-lock bag. I was not sure if it was dead, but I did not have the intestinal fortitude to find out.

For the first time in my career, I uttered the phrase, "There is potentially a live bat with the patient in acute care 4" to the emergency department staff. They looked at me in disbelief. Fleas, maggots, lice, and flying insects are routinely encountered on an average weekend and usually not a big deal, but this was a different situation. (On a side note: If you want to give health care professionals the medical heebie-jeebies, bring bed bugs into the emergency department. You will be isolated quicker than a bleeding Ebola patient with active tuberculosis.)

Despite our training and years of experience, we had no idea how to best manage this situation. The physician assistant and I decided our best course of action was to call the department of health (DOH) to get the best advice. They became alarmed at the fact that we had a bat in a healthcare setting. We were advised to place the bat in a specimen cup, put it on ice and wait for a DOH representative to pick up the animal and dispose of it with proper protocols. We obtained a specimen jar and placed the bat inside, sealed it, and then placed it on ice in a vomit basin, one of the most commonly used pieces of equipment in any emergency department.

Prior to COVID-19 pandemic protocols, we were able to eat in the emergency department. Frequently, and particularly on night shifts, staff members would often bring in snacks for the team. It makes the night shift a little more pleasant. Usually, the food will be placed in the pink vomit basins for everyone to enjoy. I always found this ironic and thought about what patients and visitors are thinking as we gorge ourselves out of containers that people vomit in (vomit, if you're lucky). This is one of the defining characteristics of an emergency department staff member: you can eat anything out of a vomit basin without thinking twice about it, oftentimes, after just being exposed to some other bodily fluid from another patient. Out of fear that someone would reach into the bat ice bath, I wrote in black magic marker: BATS ONLY, hoping that no one would stick their hands in.

Several hours passed as we were waiting for the bat to be taken, but we finally got the call. The DOH representative arrived to pick up the bat. He instructed us to carry out the bat and place it in the transport vehicle where he was waiting for us. It was an otherwise quiet night and we had a few minutes to spare, so we obliged. We placed the bat on a stretcher, with clean sheets and wheeled it out into the ambulance bay. Some staff members said their goodbyes and paid respect as it passed through the department and was loaded onto the vehicle in preparation for transport to its final destination.

In retrospect, I think these stories represent the randomness of what we deal with in the emergency department. Although some people might just say it's "a regular day in the ER," if you work in the field of emergency medicine, everyone will have their own answer to the question,

"What's the craziest thing you've ever seen?" For me, these are just a few of the stories that come to mind first. To date, I have not had any more bat funerals, but who knows what tomorrow will bring.

CONCLUSION

The stories shared by our emergency medicine physicians hopefully have provided you with greater appreciation of their dedication and sacrifice. They face daily challenges unlike any others in medicine—or any other profession, for that matter.

Before becoming executive director of Staten Island University Hospital (SIUH), I was an emergency medicine physician for over twenty years, so I have firsthand knowledge of the stressful demands of the job as well as the personal gratification it brings.

Quite simply, well-run emergency departments are environments of highly organized chaos. The professionals who work there day in and day out must learn to embrace the rigidity, but also the chaos that comes through the door—and then thrive in it.

While public health emergencies like the Covid-19 pandemic, Superstorm Sandy, and the 2003 Staten Island Ferry crash certainly stand out in the memories of caregivers at SIUH, every day brings some level of crisis to our ERs.

It's a demanding and humbling job that requires

practitioners to be prepared for anything or anyone who comes through the door, no matter how many patients they've already seen during their typically grueling shifts or how many hours of sleep they managed to get before coming to work.

They see people on what are often the worst days of their lives, struggling with life-threatening illnesses or injuries that require immediate care.

Yet, unlike many other medical professionals who specialize in a particular field of medicine, emergency physicians must be (in the words of one of our authors) "jacks of all trades," able to diagnose and treat patients who they typically have never seen before—all while worrying about all of the other things going on in the room. In no other medical specialty is there greater pressure.

As well-trained, educated, and experienced as these medical professionals may be, there are moments for which they cannot prepare. The emergency department, as one of my colleagues wrote, is a "microcosm of life," adding, "Unusual medical, social, and emotional situations leave a mark on your soul."

The practice of emergency medicine is a team sport unlike any other where the stakes are sometimes life and death. Teamwork and grit must be prioritized above all else. Few professions enjoy the same atmosphere of collaboration and comradery or experience such levels of highs and lows on a near-daily basis—feelings of triumph when lives are saved and utter dejection when they're lost.

CONCLUSION

On a personal level, nothing is more painful than delivering devastating news to grieving loved ones. Over time, these professionals learn to persevere during such dark days, but most have found themselves wondering afterwards whether they could have done anything differently that could have changed the outcome.

More than anything else, emergency medicine physicians learn the importance of maintaining their composure when stress and emotions are running high, knowing that other members of the team are looking to them for leadership. As one of my colleagues shared, the heat of the moment can impact performance, no matter how good one's muscle memory is.

Like everyone else, these professionals have families and responsibilities at home—whether it be raising children, trying to maintain strong relationships with a spouse or partner, caring for aging parents, or tackling household chores—but the stresses of their personal lives become secondary once they get to the hospital.

Like the rest of us, they also experience serious illness from time to time. As documented by one of my colleagues in these pages, the transition from caregiver to patient made him more empathetic to the plight of the dozens of people he treats every day, giving him greater appreciation for their fears and the need for compassion.

For those who enter this profession, there are many different motivations. As shared in this book, some pursue a medical career in honor or memory of a lost loved one. Others are following in the footsteps of a parent or mentor, recognizing the value of what they bring to their community and society as a whole.

If the mark of a good society is how well we care for each other, then emergency medicine professionals are the safety net of cities and towns across America—always there to serve twenty-four hours a day, seven days a week, 365 days a year.

I wanted to publish this book because I think it's important for people to understand and recognize the selfless mindset of the tens of thousands of emergency medicine physicians, nurses, and medical professionals who work in ERs around the country, including the fifty-five ER physicians at Staten Island University Hospital who treat more than 120,000 people annually.

Their heroics often extend to their personal lives, such as my colleague who saved an eighteen-month-old boy from a neighbor's pool or another who tried unsuccessfully to revive a suicide victim who jumped from a bridge overpass. They are the pillars of our community—and we owe them all a debt of gratitude.

—Brahim Ardolic, MD
Executive Director
Staten Island University Hospital

ABOUT STATEN ISLAND UNIVERSITY HOSPITAL

Staten Island University Hospital's campuses offer the leading-edge medical care one would expect from a major metropolitan hospital in a community-based atmosphere. With two campuses and 668 beds, Staten Island University Hospital is the borough's major teaching hospital and one of the New York metropolitan area's largest. After 155 years, SIUH continues to earn public and peer recognition for quality care.

SIUH is also Staten Island's largest employer with seven thousand positions. Its medical/dental staff is comprised of more than one thousand physicians and dentists who practice in over forty medical, surgical, and dental specialties and subspecialties and in a growing number of centers of care. As part of Northwell Health, SIUH has access to the vast resources of New York's largest health system, while remaining firmly entrenched and engaged in its local community.

The seventeen-acre North campus houses Staten Island's most modern emergency department, a state-of-the-art education center, and a medical arts pavilion. The South campus boasts its own emergency department and offers a range of specialty programs, including geriatric psychiatry, behavioral health care, and substance abuse services. Highly specialized units include: The Heart Institute, Florina Cancer Center, Regional Burn Center, Comprehensive Breast Cancer Center, Center for Bariatric Surgery, The Institute of Sleep Medicine, Level III Perinatal Center, and Stroke Center.

Staten Island University Hospital considers employees to be our greatest resource—and is dedicated to providing the best possible care through continuous quality improvement.